T0178915

MODERN IRIDOLOGY

MODERN IRIDOLOGY
A Holistic Guide
to Reading the Eyes

Sarah Donoghue

AEON

First published in 2023 by
Aeon Books

British Library Cataloguing in Publication Data

A C.I.P. for this book is available from the British Library

ISBN-13: 978-1-80152-052-2

Illustration by Rosemary Horne
Typeset by Medlar Publishing Solutions Pvt Ltd, India

www.aeonbooks.co.uk

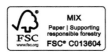

Printed and bound by CPI Group (UK) Ltd, Croydon, CR0 4YY

Imagine having a blueprint of your genetically inherited strengths and weaknesses—a comprehensive health profile that allowed you to make informed dietary and lifestyle choices that fully supported your unique constitution.

Iridology is such an invaluable tool. This book is a guide to the often-misunderstood subject—a practical manual that can easily be used by medical professionals and interested enthusiasts alike.

Complete with high quality photographs, charts, and detailed case studies, this informative handbook should be a staple on every modern healthcare practitioner's book shelf.

The aim of this book is to:

- Make iridology accessible to the busy practitioner and non-healthcare professionals with any interest and curiosity
- Compile current information into one easy-to-follow, no-nonsense, concise, essential guide
- Enable readers to safely examine the iris and make confident assessments based on the presentation of the person in front of them

- Allow readers to formulate appropriate, individualised herbal, dietary, and lifestyle interventions based on information gleaned from the iris

In short, this book takes a holistic approach to explore the subject of iridology from a scientific, physical, emotional, and spiritual perspective.

This book is for:

- Holistic healthcare providers and trained medical professionals who want to deepen their understanding and connection to their patients
- Any human being who is interested in learning about their own unique constitution to make appropriate lifestyle choices to support them in achieving vibrant wellbeing

CONTENTS

PART 1

Introduction to iridology

Introduction

"Such are the eyes; such is the body"

Hippocrates

The study of iridology is a fascinating, yet controversial one. Nobody who has ever lived (or ever will live) has the same unique iris as you. Lying somewhere between a science and a mystical art, it's been the subject of many debates among people around the world for centuries.

The development of new technology now allows anyone with a camera or magnifying tool to easily study the iris in detail. With this in mind, I felt it was high time an attempt was made to make what is a somewhat complex subject, more accessible to the growing number of people who have an increasing awareness of what it truly means to be in good health. This includes the many herbalists, acupuncturists, GPs and millions of other interested enthusiasts who are crying out for our healthcare systems to look less towards reductionist medicine and move towards a more individual, holistic approach to the way we view health and the management of disease.

My own interest in the topic began as a very small child. Having no knowledge of medicine, I was still able to intuit from my grandfather's eyes that all was not well. At age sixty-eight, he had a very common iris sign, which would now be referred to (and widely recognised by any medically trained doctor) as a cholesterol or sodium ring. The common medical term is the *arcus senilis*.

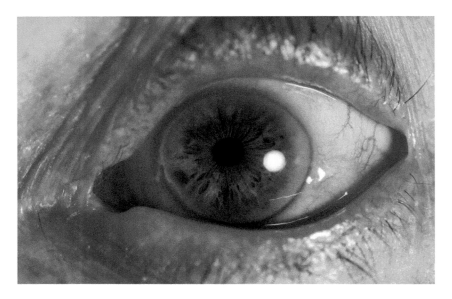

High levels of cholesterol in the arteries are visible as an opaque or foggy white ring, at the top of, or completely encircling the iris. This feature is known as the arcus senilis, and is usually found in the elderly. When observed in the eyes of patients under the age of 40, it's referred to as the arcus juvenilis, and represents an increased risk for cardiovascular disease.[1]

Some years later my grandfather developed heart related health issues, which ultimately led to his demise. I've often wondered if he had had knowledge of this quite obvious sign in his iris, could he potentially have prevented his illness from progressing?

Of course, iridology is not fortune telling, and the intention of this book is not to sensationalise or grossly exaggerate what may or may

---

[1] Akul Munjal and Evan J, Kaufman. *Arcus Senilis* (Treasure Island (FL): StatPearls Publishing, 2022).

not be seen in the iris. However, I do want to share with you what I've learned from my own clinical practice over the last thirteen years. My hope is that it will encourage you to gain deeper insights into your own wellness blue-print, and to use this information to create your own bespoke plans for optimal health. After all, iridology benefits not just those who are sick, but also those who are well. This book is therefore intended for two kinds of people—those with a health issue they wish to improve, and those who are healthy and want to stay that way.

This work is a simplified version of the rich and complex study of iridology, and is based on the format followed in the popular workshops I've taught over the last five or so years. I've been very fortunate indeed to have worked with, and learned from some of the pioneering leaders in this field, and can only hope that my own small additions to this burgeoning pot of knowledge will in some incremental way help to move the discussion forward.

In my attempts to simplify this complex topic, I've tried to do away with over complicated jargon; the goal being to make the information clear and concise, so that it may easily be applied by anyone with the right tools and mindset. The purpose of this book is not only to make the subject more accessible, but to create a desire in the reader to further explore the fascinating workings of our amazing human bodies as a hologram of the universe, of which the whole is far greater than the sum of its parts.

This practical handbook is by no means intended to serve as an exhaustive exploration of the topic, but a mere springboard to get you started on the road of discovery. I hope it will open the door of your mind just the tiniest of chinks, to the truly astounding idea that nature holds the answer to so many of our questions, if only we would take the time to stop and look.

What is iridology?

"Iridology affirms the uniqueness of each individual, and the power of the individual to manage his or her own health."[2]

Peter Jackson-Main

---

[2] Peter Jackson-Main, *Practical Iridology* (London: Carroll & Brown, 2004).

Iridology is the study of the iris (the coloured portion of the eye.) Iridologists pay close attention to the **colour, density of fibres, patterns, and markings** of the iris, to determine a person's inherited constitutional strengths and weaknesses. These observations can be used to offer valuable insights into both the genetically inherited constitution, and tendencies towards certain disease patterns of every individual. The value therefore lies in attuning people to their own bodies, with a view to encouraging them to live in harmony with their personal, natural make-up.

Iridology is not a diagnostic tool in a traditional medical sense. Its purpose is less about diagnosing specific diseases, but playing detective to reveal the underlying cause. Why does one person with stress go on to develop stomach ulcers, while another is plagued with high blood pressure?

When approached with an open and enquiring mind, iridology can provide valuable insights into the sensible measures and lifestyle interventions a person can make in order to support their unique constitution (the strengths and weaknesses you were born with.) When thoughtfully applied, this information can potentially be the difference between vibrant health and disease.

Your irides (plural of iris) are as unique and individual as your fingerprints. Even identical twins can be told apart by the differences in their iris structure. Every part of your body (and in my own personal opinion, even some aspects of your personality) are reflected within. It has been estimated that there are approximately 200 different signs which can be identified in the iris. These various patterns, colours and markings are so unique, that this biometric information is detailed enough to distinguish you from every other human being on the planet.

The structure of the iris stems from the neural pathways of the brain. In fact, it's the only part of the body where these nerve fibres can be clearly viewed. Early pioneers believed that these nervous reflexes pertained to corresponding organs of the body, hence the interest in a person's eyes as a helpful diagnostic tool.

As I hope to demonstrate, naturopaths, herbalists, and in fact any other healthcare professional can use this information to provide lifestyle advice, formulate bespoke prescriptions, and offer individual treatment protocols as a form of preventative and corrective medicine. This is known as bio-iridology.[3]

---

[3] James Colton and Sheelagh Colton, *Iridology—Health Analysis & Treatments from the Iris of the Eye* (UK: Element books, 1996), 1.

Fact vs fiction: what iridology can (and can't) tell you

A quick Google search for Iridology will pull up a wide array of videos, bold claims, and often bizarre facts. I guarantee you will also find a substantial selection of articles claiming it is outright quackery. Let's set the record straight about what iridology is and (more importantly) is not.

Iridology CANNOT:

- Tell you if you are pregnant. Conception is a normal healthy process and not a disease.
- Diagnose viral infections such as Covid (although it remains to be seen if traces or "miasms"[4] of the damage caused by this novel situation will show up in the eyes of future generations). Most common childhood infections (e.g. Chicken pox, the common cold), are transient situations, and as such, do not show up in the iris.
- Diagnose cancer (although it may provide indications of inherited energy weakness within the various tissues, which could make that site a potential area of concern for any number of pathological processes to unfold.)
- Tell you if you have candida, toxicity, or a build up of heavy metals in your body. (Although there is still some debate around this topic, it is my view that further studies need to be done.)
- Determine if healing is taking place in any organ.[5]

Iridology CAN:

- Offer clues about the health issues you are most susceptible to based on your unique constitution inherited at birth.
- Offer insights into genetic traits that can be strengthened or improved with nutrition and good lifestyle habits.
- Highlight certain personality traits *to some extent*. This is known as emotional iridology or Rayid iris interpretation, and is the branch of iridology which is most fervently criticized by its opponents.

---

[4] Miasm—a weakness or mark left behind after physical disease which can be transmitted down the generational chain.

[5] Although the fore-founders of Iridology believed they were able to see lines form in the eye as healing took place, modern advancements in photography and digital imaging suggest this does not actually happen. The fact remains that for the most part, the iris structure is determined at birth and does not change or alter over a person's lifetime.

The long and short of it is that since the dawn of time, people have made observations about the human body that allow us to intuit certain facts about them. Should we choose to take heed of the signs that nature mirrors back to us (the lustre of one's skin, the light in one's eyes, the texture of a person's fingernails,) we can tentatively begin to make informed assessments about their current state of wellbeing.

Iridology takes this one step further by using data collected over time to create a reliable (but at times imperfect) system. In short, the goal is to use these iris observations to better understand the inherent strengths and weaknesses we are born with. Not only does this offer an exciting possibility for us to gain knowledge of how to take better care of ourselves, but an opportunity to invest in the health of future generations.

The iridology problem

Although iridology of a sorts was at one time taught in medical schools, many modern orthodox practitioners are quick to dismiss or even ridicule the study. This is despite the fact there are many signs visible in the eyes that are universally recognised by the allopathic medical profession, and are known to correlate with certain conditions.

Here is a small selection to illustrate the point:

Anaemia

Iron deficiency can prevent blood from carrying sufficient oxygen to the eye tissues. If you pull down your lower eyelid, the inside layer should be a healthy red colour. If it is very pale (or even yellow), this is usually an indicator of low iron levels. Dark circles under the eyes are another sign that oxygen may not be being adequately delivered to the tissues.

In iridology, chronic anaemia can appear as a bright blue ring around the outer edge of the iris. It can be visible in either the upper or lower portion of the eye (or both), and is easily viewed with the naked eye. This phenomenon is caused by the white of the eye (the sclera) invading the iris.

If any of these signs are observed either by an Iridologist or other medical practitioner, it would be prudent to question the patient about their energy levels, mood, and diet, and if possible, refer them for a blood test to confirm their iron levels are within the normal range.

Brushfield's spots (see also lymphatic rosary)

Brushfield's spots are small, white, yellow or greyish/brown spots found towards the outer edge of the iris. These spots are named after the physician Thomas Brushfield who first described them in his thesis in 1924.[6] Anyone can be born with Brushfield's spots, but interestingly, it is a common feature in persons born with Down's syndrome.[7]

The sign appears to be more common in blue eyed individuals. However, some iridologists think this may be due to the fact they are more difficult to observe in people with darker iris pigmentation, which obscures the feature. In iridology books, you may also see this sign described as the lymphatic rosary.[8]

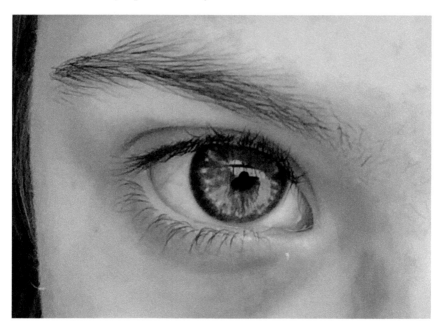

Brushfield spots are visible towards the outer edge of the iris and usually appear in pairs. Iridologists refer to this iris sign as the lymphatic rosary.

---

[6] Lavinia Postolache and Cameron F. Parsa, "Brushfield Spots and Wölfflin Nodules Unveiled in Dark Irides Using near-Infrared Light," *Scientific Reports* 8, no. 1 (2018). https://doi.org/10.1038/s41598-018-36348-6.

[7] Danielle Ledoux, "Vision and Down Syndrome," published 2022, *National Down Syndrome Society*. https://ndss.org/resources/vision-down-syndrome

[8] Refer to information on the lymphatic rosary on Pg 74.

Liver disease

Jaundice is caused by the build-up of a yellow substance called bilirubin, which turns the skin and whites of the eyes yellow. It is often a sign of a problem with the liver, gallbladder or pancreas, and may be an indicator of serious health conditions such as liver disease.[9] As such, this is outside of the remit of the iridologist and it is recommended for the patient to be immediately referred to their GP.

Thyroid issues

Hypothyroidism (an underactive thyroid) can sometimes cause swelling around the eyes and a loss of the hairs in the outer part of the eyebrows. If hypothyroidism develops after treatment for Graves' disease (the most common form of *overactive* thyroid,) it can cause a problem known as Graves' ophthalmopathy. About 30% of people with Graves' disease show some signs of Graves' ophthalmopathy, symptoms of which include visibly protruding eyeballs, a gritty sensation in the eyes, light sensitivity and double vision.[10]

Thyroid eye disease is a condition in which the eye muscles, eyelids, tear glands and fatty tissues behind the eye become inflamed. This can cause the eyes and eyelids to become red, swollen and uncomfortable. In some cases, the eyes can be pushed forward, giving the person the appearance of having staring or bulging eyes.[11]

I hope I've demonstrated that even at this surface level, it must be agreed that the body has many different ways to alert us when all is not well. Despite observational skills being a crucial element of the training of medical practitioners, a quick trawl of the internet will show that a large number of people are still reluctant to accept the value of exploring the subject of iridology with an open, enquiring mind.

---

[9] The National Library of Medicine, "Jaundice Causes", MedlinePlus, 2022. https://med-lineplus.gov/ency/article/007491.htm

[10] Mayo Clinic, "Graves' disease—Patient care & health information," 2022. *Mayo Foundation for Medical Education and Research (MFMER)* https://www.mayoclinic.org/diseases-conditions/graves-disease/symptoms-causes/syc-20356240

[11] British Thyroid Foundation, "Thyroid Eye Disease," Revised 2021. https://www.btf-thyroid.org/thyroid-eye-disease-leaflet

Claims that the lack of evidence for signs correlating to illness must by definition render the entire subject baseless in science are unhelpful. As we shall see, there are a large number of observations (other than the obvious markings and colourations), that are invaluable in making a sensible and helpful assessment of the person in front of you.

> *"Here is the Sign—Where is the Ulcer?"*[12]
>
>   Ignaz Von Péczely

The difference between iris markings and presenting clinical findings has always been a problematic conundrum for iridologists. Over the years it has (and still remains), a seriously divisive stumbling block when it comes to validating the practice of iridology.

"Hic signum ubi ulcus?"—Here is the sign, where is the ulcer?—is a quote made famous by Ignaz Von Péczely, a Hungarian doctor, widely credited as being one of the first people to propose iridology be taken seriously as a medical science. His entire life was devoted to pondering this question, and was a sticking point that haunted the so-called "Father of Iridology" until his dying day.

The burning question that still divides proponents of iridology and skeptics is:

> *Does an iris marking indicate a current health problem or a latent condition?*

This has always been a bone of contention among critics of iridology, and as we shall later see, was even more of a challenge for the very first pioneers of the study.

Let's address the importance of this question.

As I hope I've already outlined, iridology is not so much about identifying the symptom and offering reductionist diagnoses, but uncovering the root cause of disease by taking into account the individual's unique inherited make-up. In this respect, we are taking care of the person as well as the presenting problem.

---

[12] Emil Schlegel, *Die Augendiagnose des Dr. Ignaz von Péczely*, 1887, reprint, (Antique Reprints, 2016).

Being ill and not knowing why is unfortunately (and increasingly), an extremely distressing reality for many people for whom expensive tests and medications haven't helped (I include in this the vast and bamboozling array of vitamin, herbal and nutritional supplements currently available on the market.) It is my own personal belief that if a person is armed with knowledge about how to live in harmony with their inherited constitution from the get-go, then markings in the iris offer a helpful opportunity to serve as *cautionary warning signs,* rather than indelible imprints of a forgone conclusion.

People who are skeptical about the study of iridology often demand "proof" of outcome. I myself have been put to the uncomfortable test of assessing a person's health based purely on a photograph, without having any prior knowledge of the patient's case history. This a very reductionist view and put quite simply, *is not the way iridology works.*

Any orthodox medical practitioner will tell you that the art of diagnosis itself is wide open to interpretation. If that were not the case, every lump, bump, and runny nose would have to be subject to a battery of tests, which themselves would be open to all manner of interpretation; not all of which would reveal the same underlying cause of the problem. In his book, *Leechcraft,* Stephen Pollington[13] quotes a BBC Radio 4 programme[14] in which the claim was made that as little as ten percent of modern medical treatments are evidence based, but rather based on the practitioner's own knowledge experiences, preferences, and intuition.

As a clinical herbalist I have encountered many people in my office who have arrived there being unable to receive an adequate diagnosis from their own GP. It is for this reason that I firmly believe that *if used in a sensitive way and in conjunction with a detailed case history,* iridology has the potential to offer valuable information about *predispositions to certain ailments* making prevention possible, as well as offering a viable method of getting to the root cause of what is going on.

In my book, this makes iridology a very valuable tool indeed for every person on the planet.

---

[13] Stephen Pollington, *Leechcraft—Early English Charms, Plantlore & Healing* (Cambridgeshire: Anglo-Saxon Books, 2011) 16.
[14] BBC Radio 4. Sunday 11th January 1998.

Iridology pioneers

"The iris dictates the prescription"

Pastor E Felke

As the main goal of this book is to serve as a practical manual, it is not my intention to go into great detail about the history and background of iridology here. Although a fascinating topic, there are already a number of good books that tell the tale of iridology's history in much more detail for those of you who have an interest.[15]

However, it would be remiss not to briefly mention some of the main protagonists in the story. This isn't just because they're fabulously interesting characters, but because they personally inspire me to want to take up the mantle where they left off.

Here are a few of my favourite iridologists (in no particular order).

Jean-Nicolas Corvisart des Marets (1755–1821)

In 1801, during a dinner reception, Corvisart was introduced to General Napoleon Bonaparte. The General's wife Josephine asked "To what disease do you think the General is most likely to be exposed?" "To a disease of the heart," replied Corvisart. "Have you written a book on that?" asked Napoleon. "No but I intend to publish one soon." "Then lose no time, we will speak on that later."[16]

Jean-Nicolas Corvisart-Desmarets was a pioneer in cardiology, and responsible for the popularisation of the chest percussion technique.[17] He later became Bonaparte's personal physician.

He began his career in the poor neighbourhoods of Paris. Unlike his colleagues who focused their attention on dead people and their demise, his special area of interest was in recognising diseases from his living patient's presenting signs and symptoms. He was an outspoken

---

[15] See further resources section at the end of this book.
[16] Marianna Karamanou, Charalambos Vlachopoulos, Christodoulos Stefanadis & George Androutsos, "Professor Jean-Nicolas Corvisart des Marets (1755–1821): Founder of modern cardiology", *Hellenic journal of cardiology: HJC/Hellēnikē kardiologikē epitheōrēsē.* 51 (2010): 290–3. https://www.researchgate.net/publication/45281897_Professor_Jean-Nicolas_Corvisart_des_Marets_1755-1821_Founder_of_modern_cardiology
[17] Karamanou, "Corvisart des Marets", 290–3. https://www.researchgate.net/publication/45281897_Professor_Jean-Nicolas_Corvisart_des_Marets_1755-1821_Founder_of_modern_cardiology

man with a firm belief that every person was unique, and that disease developed due to the body's individuality, rather than its generalised consistency. His approach was to observe his patient's presenting symptoms, rather than adhering to a set checklist of how a certain disease must manifest.

This was very avant-garde for his day, and in stark contrast with the prevailing view of the time which was that, unless faced with an unknown catalyst, the natural state of the human body was to remain in consistent health. An unhealthy body was presumed to be the result of either an imbalance, or an external pathogenic cause. Corvisart's belief in individual variation was an abrupt challenge to this assumption.

Today it is widely accepted that science is based on observation. In this respect, Covisart can be credited with making a huge contribution to the study of pathological anatomy.

Ignaz Von Pescely (1822–1911)

Ignaz Von Peczely was a Hungarian doctor who is widely credited as being the "Father of Iridology."[18] The story goes, that at as very young boy he was fond of animals and yearned for a pet of his own. The family home was quite close to a forest, and one day while out walking, he stumbled across an injured owl in distress. Ignaz tried to wrap the bird in his coat, but as it struggled, it's leg became entangled and was further injured. Ignaz was distraught. Fearing that he may have inadvertently harmed the bird, he decided to take it home and try to nurse it back to health.

Now owls have very large eyes, and it's reported that Ignaz had observed a white cloud in one eye (on the same side as the injured leg), which over the weeks turned into a black spot and eventually vanished to an imperceptible thin white line. Ignaz thought this so unusual, it sparked an obsession that was to last a lifetime. He began keeping records of the various "signs" he noticed in the eyes of the people he met. He soon gained a reputation for having an astounding ability to read a person's health from their eyes. Before long, people began flocking from far and wide to consult with him. Whatever the origins of this story (which have inevitably been embellished as time has gone by), the details of his later life are well documented.[19]

---

[18] Guild of Naturopathic Iridologists International, "The History of Iridology," 2023, https://www.gni-international.org/the-history-of-iridology/
[19] Colton, "Iridology", 26–27.

In his youth he was involved in the uprising of 1848 and was sent to prison for being an activist. Not having much to occupy his time, he began to study his fellow inmates, making drawings of his observations and keeping records of their health. He was surprised to find many correlations between their wellbeing and the information he recorded from their eyes.

Upon his release, he trained as a medical doctor, graduating with honours from Budapest University. This is when he began studying the iris in earnest. The surgical wards offered many opportunities to study the eyes of his patients both before and after their operations. Not only did he keep records of the eyes of his living patients, he also researched markings in the eyes of bodies in the hospital morgue. This provided a unique opportunity to correlate his findings with the diseases the people had died from. Over many years he collated meticulous notes which he used to compile the first iris chart.

In 1881 he published his work, *The Discovery in Natural History and Medical Science: A Guide to the Study and Diagnosis from the Eye*, which gained him international fame. However, he was widely criticised for this work, and his many confrontations with his medical colleagues eventually sent him into a spiral of depression. Ridicule of his work reached a pinnacle at a medical conference in London where permission to publish his lecture was openly denounced. This was the final nail in the coffin, and he became totally disheartened and gave up. He was never able to get over the stumbling block of the difference between the iris markings and his clinical findings, which he made with only the help of a 2x magnification lens and was a source of further ridicule.

Despite his tragic end, it's widely held that the work carried out by this forward-thinking man, provided the foundations for others to take up the mantle. It was due to his pioneering work that the scientific study of iridology was born.

Joseph Deck (1914–1990)

Joseph Deck had the ambitious goal to one day make iridology an accepted practice in mainstream medicine. He was a huge fan of Ignaz Von Pescely, and spent many years of his life trying to vindicate his findings.

In 1935 he invited leading Iridologists of the time to attend a conference, with the aim of finally solving the mystery of the question that had plagued Von Pescely all of his life;

Does a marking indicate a current problem or a latent health condition?

Unfortunately, as nobody came forward to fund his project, he soon found he was the only person willing to work on the problem. Before long it became apparent just how frustrating this mystery must have been for poor Ignaz Von Pescely. Undeterred, Joseph Deck eventually had a breakthrough. In 1950 he examined a well-known professor of medicine and found a marking in the stomach and left-hand side of the upper abdomen. He made detailed notes and drawings, and explained his findings to the doctor who remarked that he had no known problems in this area.

Eleven years later, an unexpected perforation of the stomach occurred, which required the doctor to have a partial gastrectomy. After the successful operation, Deck once again approached the doctor in the hope he would now have a well-respected ally to back his claims. To his horror and dismay, the doctor proclaimed he had no recollection of being examined by Joseph, even going as far as to say that he firmly believed that iris diagnosis had no value for the medical profession.

Fuelled by rage, Joseph Deck was more determined than ever to prove his theory. He began looking at old cases and focusing on certain markings that did in fact manifest at a later date. His self-published work, *The Fundamentals of Iridology*,[20] was published in German in 1965, but his endeavours were never officially recognised. He died in 1992.

Like all pioneers, these are people who had the courage to raise their head above the parapet for the purpose of scientific enquiry. In common with many people who possess a forward-thinking mindset, they were highly ridiculed for their ideas, which although imperfect, were certainly ahead of their time. Hindsight is a wonderful thing. With the advancement of medical science, photographic equipment and a much better understanding of the body as a holistic system, we now have the luxury of revisiting this knowledge with a view to verifying and refining the study. Iridology is not an exact science, but just because it isn't perhaps as commercially viable as some of the (often very expensive) investigative medical tests currently on the market, this doesn't mean we should relegate the entire subject to the rubbish bin. Perhaps now is the perfect moment to use advancements in our knowledge to "fill in the gaps" and continue on where these inspirational pioneers left off.

---

[20] Joseph Deck. *Fundamentals of Iridology.* 1st Edition, (Etlingen: Self-published, 1965).

PART 2

Looking at the iris competently and safely

Buying the right tools

When I first began to study iridology as a student, the cost for specialist equipment was way beyond my financial means. This certainly didn't prevent me from picking up a cheap hand-held magnifier, which I used for a number of years before I was able to afford more technical equipment. I still have that magnifier. I often use it when I need to make a quick assessment, or in times when taking a photograph simply isn't practical. Just because they're relatively cheap and easy to pick up, doesn't mean that they're not valuable tools. They're certainly adequate enough for a hobbyist to gain some really valuable insights when first starting out.

Hand held magnifiers

A magnifying glass with a light loupe and around 10x magnification (the kind a stamp collector might use,) is sufficient to begin with. I have experimented using magnifiers both with and without battery operated lights, and the general consensus when practicing with different equipment at various workshops has always been that a light is best.

Examining the iris safely

Eyeball to eyeball contact is a primal communication system that has always existed between humans. Having the privilege to experience an up-close encounter with a person's iris is about as close to their soul as one can get. Although it can feel exciting to see a person's iris up close, always remember to follow rule number one—don't be a space invader! The comfort of the client must always remain your first priority. For this reason, I always recommend looking at the person's eye from the side. A head on confrontation a few millimetres from a person's face is a very disconcerting and off-putting experience. Try to be aware that you are entering someone's personal space, and they are revealing intimate information about their physical wellbeing to you.

Children in particular can be very sensitive about what comes close to their eyes. A good way to get around this is to let them handle the magnifier or torch. I often ask them to look at their parent or guardian's eye and see if they can find a Cornish pixie! This is usually enough to gain their confidence up to a point where they are happy for you to take a closer look.

Have the person look straight ahead (they may want to rest their head on the back of a chair), and look forward with a still gaze. It is helpful to give them a point to look at (a wandering eye is impossible to examine), before trying to discern the main signs. Avoid having the patient stare into the light for long periods of time. Ten seconds is about the maximum you should have in mind when making your examination. Give the person breaks. Move away and write something down, let the eye relax and then come back again if need be.

Most importantly of all, *be sure to examine both eyes*. You would be amazed at the number of amateur iridologists who make their observations on only one iris. Humans are not cyclops! As we'll shortly see, there are an amazing number of differences between the two eyes, and only examining one may mean missing some vital clue that is crucially important in the persons health profile.

Photographing the iris—how to do it

We are fortunate to live in an age of incredible technology. Unlike the days of Ignaz Von Pescely, digital cameras, iriscopes, and other high spec optical instruments allow us to gather, compare, and assess images of the iris in great detail.

Taking a photograph is often a safer, less intrusive, and more useful way of studying the iris, and has a number of clear advantages over using a traditional hand-held magnifier.

Despite the fact that we look at ourselves in the mirror every day, most people have never taken the time to take a close up look at their own eyes. The most satisfying part of my workshops is seeing the reactions of people who are properly seeing their eyes for the very first time. It really is incredible to see the excitement on the face of a person who has just discovered something completely new about themselves.

Never underestimate the power of a photograph. Not only is it an incredibly humbling experience to see your own eyes in such detail, it's often the trigger for a person to volunteer all manner of intimate details they may never have thought important, (or even considered volunteering) when they first walked into your office.

Using a photograph to discuss one's constitutional health is a very empowering tool. An on-the-spot analysis using a hand-held magnifier can actually have the opposite effect. The invasive presence of a stranger holding a bright light to your eye is a naturally uncomfortable experience. Not only does having a picture allow the person to see what *you* are seeing, it avoids having a limited time frame in which to make rapid assessments of what's in front of you.

Advantages of taking a photograph

- Taking a photograph allows you the luxury of going away and assessing the iris in more detail. You have time to look closely at the markings and refer to an iris chart if needed.
- Taking multiple pictures allows you to compensate for any lighting conditions that may affect the nature of the image.
- It eliminates the amount of light exposure to the eye, which may be uncomfortable and intrusive for the client.
- It engages the client, who will often offer up important information, which may be invaluable in formulating a treatment plan.
- It allows you to keep a record of the iris and compare any follow up photographs.
- It allows you to build up a library of cases you can use as reference points, or to discover new information that can be added to the pot.

Using a digital camera

To take the best photos for your reading, set your camera to *macro* and try, if possible, to use natural, daytime, indoor light, and use a flash.

Set the size of the photo for a higher resolution, with a minimum of 2.5M (2208 × 1248). 4.5M (2784 × 1568) is best.

- Set the camera to macro setting.
- Increase the resolution to 4.5M (2784 × 1568).
- Turn on the flash.
- Adjust the light so that the image in the view finder is crisp and clear. Stand sideways from any window (facing the window will cause glare).
- Keep the eye close to the camera. On macro setting, you can be approximately 4–5 inches away from the lens.
- If it is comfortable for the sitter, ask them to hold their upper and lower eyelids open to make sure that the entire iris is visible.
- Use the zoom feature to see the iris clearly.
- Take one photo of each iris at a time, followed by a quick burst. That way you will have several pictures to choose from when it's time to make your assessment.
- Check the photos for red eye; otherwise turn on "red eye reduction" and try again.
- Finally, take a quick flick through your pictures to ensure you have what you need. There is nothing worse than sitting down to make your assessment and realising that your pictures are not clear enough for your needs.

When taking photographs, it's important to remember the effect that the light has both on the pupil and muscle tone of the eye. Upon first glance, you will notice that the pupil initially contracts and becomes smaller in an attempt to reduce the amount of light entering the eye. To compensate for this (and to achieve an accurate picture), give the person a few moments to adjust to the light. Don't make them stare at it for so long it's blinding, but for just enough time to allow the pupil to naturally settle before committing to taking your photo.

This is another reason why it is vital to take more than one photograph. By doing this you can be sure that any visible markings are what you think they are. You'd be surprised how much contractions can distort the iris, changing both the shape and nature of the markings and signs present.

Should you be in a position to invest in equipment there are a number of options available:

- Digital cameras with a macro lens
- Iriscope

I've included a number of practical resources (along with a list of reputable suppliers) in the reference section at the end of this book.

PART 3

First impressions

Practitioners of Traditional Chinese Medicine (TCM) have long understood the value of observing their patients using a number of different diagnostic techniques. These include feeling the nature of the pulse, examining the tongue, and noting a person's general appearance (including the quality and lustre of the hair, skin, and eyes).

I've already alluded to the fact that this practice appears to have fallen out of favour here in the West, but the health of our patients would be so much better served if we would only take the time to hone these skills, and encourage practitioners of all disciplines to become more inquisitive and do the same.

As an absolute beginner, and with no prior knowledge of iridology, there's a lot you can do by way of employing basic observational skills (alongside your intuition), to gain crucial insights into the nature of your client's current health situation. The following section is designed to get you thinking about a person's nature and how their personality, behaviours, and traits can allow you to glean information about their current health status.

Observation skills

Honing your skills of observation in everyday life is an essential tool for the aspiring iridologist.

As a college student, my friend and I would often play the "constitution game" by trying to guess people's iris type (and likely personality), on first impression. Although hardly scientific, we would often be pleasantly surprised by the number of "hits" we would get. After three years of study, we became quite good at it, to the point where we joked about setting up some sort of dating service based on our observations. I'm not suggesting you try to assess every person you pass on the street, but making mental notes about the people you meet, and applying your knowledge to those you already know quite well is a really good way to practice "getting your eye in" (pardon the pun!) and making educated guesses about the personality traits and ailments that certain iris types may have in common.

Before we get into more specific detail about the colour, structure, and markings of the iris, there are a few simple things you can do to begin training your eye. With practice, you'll soon get used to looking at eyes and forming some simple opinions about the person who owns them.

Shen

Interestingly, disharmony of Shen manifests as lacklustre eyes.

In Traditional Chinese Medicine (TCM,) the concept of shen is literally translated as "root of the spirit." Along with qi (life force) and jing (essence), shen (spirit) is considered to be one of the three treasures that are essential for life. Shen embodies consciousness, emotions, and thought, and presides over all activities that take place on the mental, spiritual, and creative plane. It is through shen that we're able to understand the nature of the universe around us, and radiate our own inner essence out into the world.

We've all seen people who seem to have lost "the light in their eyes." This often happens when a person is sad, depressed, suffering, or in emotional pain. In our modern Western culture, it would seem almost laughable for a person to go and visit their GP because they had noticed the light in their eyes had gone out, yet medical practitioners from other traditions would view this as a serious matter in need of urgent attention.

The dimming of the light in one's eyes is a sign that "the master has left the house". In short, there's no-one home—the spirit has left the body. TCM would treat such a condition with acupuncture, nourishing herbs, and activities like tai-chi or qi gong that encouraged the spirit to become grounded and return back to the body.

No special training is needed to see when a person is feeling like this. However, in our busy world, how often do we take the time to look (or heaven forbid, ask) about this crucial sign? I've seen many people in my practice who have come for herbal support for all manner of ailments, yet failed to mention that they're suffering in their emotional life. They don't write about it on their intake form, and even if asked directly, will say they're fine—yet the light in their eyes is gone. Failure to pick up on this basic sign and omitting to evaluate the person's emotional wellbeing could mean all the effort you put into your carefully crafted formula or diet plan is likely to go to waste.

The pupils

After observing the general nature of the eye, the next thing to pay close attention to is the size, position, and movement of the pupil.

Pupil size

You may be surprised to learn that the size of a person's pupil can tell you a great deal about their personality, outlook on life and how they're feeling. For example, how do you react when meeting a person with very contracted, small pupils? What would be your initial impression? Which adjectives might you use to describe this person's demeanour? Would you say they had "beady eyes?" Might you consider them to be sharp eyed, suspicious, wary, closed off? Now do the same with people with large pupils. Do they seem open, frightened, vague, flamboyant, dreamy?

Of course, the size of a person's pupils can fluctuate depending on their mood, for example if they're surprised or feeling anxious etc. However, some people have naturally larger or smaller pupils, which can also be a reflection of their normal constitutional tendencies.

Why do some people have naturally smaller or larger pupils than others?

Pupil size is related to the functioning of the autonomic nervous system, so named because it works autonomously—i.e. without any conscious effort on our behalf.

It can be broadly categorised into two complimentary systems; sympathetic and parasympathetic. The job of these two systems is to balance one another out, so we can respond appropriately to the regular demands of everyday life.

The natural way of things is for our nervous system to fluctuate between the two. However, some people can become fixed in one mode, which eventually becomes their default state. It can be useful to determine if the person in front of you has slipped into one state or the other (this can happen in cases of trauma for example where people are locked in flight, fight or freeze mode), and if so, formulate an appropriate treatment protocol to help gently bring them back into balance.

The parasympathetic nervous system is located in between the spinal cord and the medulla (the bottom-most part of your brain.) It's main purpose it to stop your body from overworking and restore you to a calm and composed state. In this respect, it can be thought of as being responsible for "rest and digest." It does this by doing things like slowing down your heart rate, or signalling to the digestive system to secrete the enzymes needed for breaking down food. When the parasympathetic nervous system is dominant, the pupils naturally contract and appear smaller.

On the other hand, **the sympathetic nervous system** is called into action whenever it's time to jump into action. It responds to potential threats by speeding up your heart rate and widening your pupils. This allows in maximum light and information, preparing you to immediately launch into survival mode and be ready to deal with any potential threats.

Small pupils

It's a fair assessment to say that people whose pupils are generally smaller than average are mostly under the influence of the parasympathetic nervous system.[21]

---

[21] Jackson-Maine, *Practical Iridology*, 21.

People with small pupils may be naturally introverted, and are often less likely to be motivated to engage with the physical world. When out of balance, they can become closed off to new ideas and situations. From an emotional perspective, we might say that the person is having difficulty allowing light, ideas, or even other people into their energetic field.

Small pupils are often a sign that the person is self-protective—this trait is most often found in combination with a silk type constitution[22]. These people tend to have a need to be in control, and use this as a coping strategy to allay anxiety and incubate a feeling of safety. People with this as their dominant constitutional type may have difficulty trusting others, or releasing their emotions in order to move forward in life.

Small pupils can also indicate over-tense muscle tone. People with unusually small pupils may suffer with issues such as tension headaches, muscular aches and pains, or stiff joints. A lack of movement can compound this tendency, and so they should be encouraged to find ways to include more physical activity in their day as a way of expending any excess energy and relieving pent up stress.

If a client with very small pupils walks into your office, you may want to focus your questions around the following:

- How do they express their emotions?
- How is their digestive system functioning?
- Do they have problems eliminating? (For example, regular bowel motions, clogged pores, pent up emotions etc.)
- Do they have any eating disorders?
- How do they normally deal with stress?
- Do they experience frequent headaches?
- Do they suffer with joint pain or experience other musculoskeletal issues?
- Do they suffer from a lack of enthusiasm for life, or have a history of depression?

Due to this person's inherent nature, be aware of sensitivity with your questioning technique. Watch their response (which may in fact tell you more than they actually say). Try to get them to open up about why they

---

[22] See Part 5—Structure and inherited disposition. Pg 45. The silk iris.

might have found themselves in your office, and if any emotional issues might be impacting their physical health.

Large pupils

On the contrary, people with large, very wide-open pupils (larger than one quarter of the diameter of the iris) may be considered to be much more open and engaged with the world. Children for example are often thought of as being "wide eyed," their curious nature is to be naturally open to learning all they can about the world around them.

People with large pupils tend to be more active and outgoing than the introverted type. From a personality viewpoint, they're often creative, open to new ideas and situations, but aren't always aware of how to maintain appropriate boundaries in order to protect their vital energy reserves.

People with larger pupils are more likely to be under the influence of the sympathetic nervous system, which is primarily responsible for the fight or flight response. The danger for these people is that because so much of their energy is consumed with life (oftentimes spent in a hyper vigilant state), they quickly become exhausted. In short, they give away so much of their energy there are never enough reserves left over in the tank.

In extreme cases, constant overstimulation of the adrenal glands culminates in actual physical exhaustion, leading to burnout or conditions such as ME. Treatment of the nervous system and adrenals is essential to help restore the person's ability to switch off, relax, and establish a healthy routine for restorative sleep.

If a client with very dilated pupils walks into your office, you may want to think about asking them questions along the lines of the following:

- How do they relax?
- Do they have high blood pressure?
- Do they regularly use stimulants like caffeine to keep going when they know they should rest?
- What is their sleep pattern like?
- How stressful is their job? Do they enjoy working in a high-pressure environment?
- Do they use alcohol or drugs as a coping mechanism?
- Do they have any addictions or compulsions? (Over-eating or over-exercising etc.)

Different-sized pupils

Although quite rare, people can sometimes present with different sized pupils. There are a number of serious health issues that might cause this to happen.[23]

- Ask about any head injuries—concussion or spinal illnesses such as meningitis can cause differentiation in pupil size.
- Tumours can press on the optic nerve.
- High fevers can affect pupil size.
- In some instances, when one pupil is noticeably smaller than the other it can indicate that the person is having a stroke.

In short, differences in pupil size should always be considered a red flag, and as such, need to be properly investigated. Don't waste time—refer the person to their GP without delay.

Sanpaku eyes

"The eye is a sign of great vitality of the rising sun. He who has this eye doesn't know fear or insecurity. All babies are like this. However, if a taxi driver is Sanpaku, it is better to avoid a ride in his car. Watch your opponent with whom you enter into negotiation because he is tricky."

George Ohsawa

The concept of Sanpaku eyes is derived from the tradition of Oriental physiognomy (face reading,) made popular by George Ohsawa in his 1971 book on the topic of Macrobiotics.[24]

Sanpaku is loosely translated as "the three whites" and refers to the white space (sclera) when it is visible either above or below the iris.

---

[23] It is also prudent to be aware that variation in pupil size may also occur with the use of certain drugs. Opiates and other tranquilizers tend to cause contraction of the pupils, whereas stimulating drugs such as amphetamines and hallucinogens result in a wide-eyed appearance. The size of the pupils may in some cases be related to a person's medication. Again, this is another reason why case taking plays a crucial role in a professional consultation.

[24] George Ohsawa, *Macrobiotics—An Invitation to Health & Happiness,* 6th Edition. (California: George Ohsawa Macrobiotic Foundation, 1984).

Although the concept of Sanpaku is somewhat controversial, it does have some basis in medical fact.

In Western medicine, this is known as lower or inferior scleral show and can be an indicator of a number of recognised medical conditions, such as endocrine imbalance (for example an overactive thyroid) or physical trauma.

According to the theory, if the sclera is visible beneath the iris, then this represents a physical imbalance in the body. It is sometimes seen in people who consume a lot of alcohol or over indulge in sugar. Conversely, if the upper sclera is visible, it may be an indicator of mental or emotional imbalance.

The theory became so popular, it was even mentioned in a song featured on the 1973 John Lennon album Mind Games.[25]

Checklist

Now you have some idea about what to look for during your first encounter with a client. Below is a checklist of factors to take into consideration *before* you get out your torch to conduct an examination:

- Is the eye clear and bright?
- Is the person focused on you or looking around?
- Does the person appear distracted? Do they have an intense stare?
- Do they have a "sparkle" in their eyes?
- Do they have noticeably large or small pupils?
- Do they have bulging eyes, or any visible white sclera above or below the iris?
- Is there any discolouration of the sclera?
- Is there any redness, puffiness or dark circles under the eyes?
- Are there any red flag signs you need to be aware of?
- What is your *general impression* of this person's demeanour?

---

[25] John Lennon, *"Aisumasen (I'm Sorry)"*, July–August 1973, track 3, side 1 on *Mind Games*, Apple, 1973, vinyl.

Exercise

Spend some time honing your observation skills by looking more closely at the eyes of the people you meet in your everyday life. What are your initial impressions? How accurate are they?

If you're feeling inspired, I encourage you to check out an amazing piece of performance art entitled *The Artist is Present*.[26] The film by Marina Abramovic involves her sitting in a chair and gazing into the eyes of strangers. Over the course of nearly three months, for eight hours a day, she met the gaze of 1,000 strangers, many of whom were moved to tears. It's truly remarkable to see the incredible power that simply looking at someone's eyes can have. The unspoken communication between the two sitters really is extra-ordinary.

Although I don't recommend staring at strangers in the street, paying closer attention to the people you encounter is an excellent way to gain more intuitive, nuanced insights which go beyond scientific explanations and uncover different aspects of the personality which may be having a direct impact on their wellbeing.[27]

---

[26] *Marina Abramovic: The Artist is Present,* directed by Matthew Akers. (Show of Force, 2012), film.

[27] If the topic of emotional Iridology appeals to you, I would certainly recommend taking a deeper dive into the world of rayid (the topic of which a whole book could be devoted). Along with new studies in the field of behavioural iridology, rayid offers a whole new dimension to what we can glean in regards to the deeper aspects of a person's personality traits and psyche. References to further recommended reading can be found in the resources section at the end of this book.

PART 4

Constitution—what the colour of your eyes says about you

> *"All man's diseases originate in his constitution. It is necessary that his constitution should be known if we wish to know his diseases."*
>
> Paracelsus

What can you learn from the colour of your eyes?

Now that you've made your initial assessments, it's time to look deeper and begin to make some more refined observations. The next obvious step is to determine the person's eye colour, which isn't as easy as it first may seem.

Focusing on the iris colour is good practice for beginner iridologists, as this alone will provide a good starting point for discussion. Many people are often surprised when they first see their eyes up close up to learn that they are not in fact a true brown or blue eyed individual, and that the range of colours that can be perceived in the iris is really quite spectacular.

Until you become more confident in finding your way around the eye, focusing on the patient's eye colour is a good entry point to gain valuable insights into suitable treatment protocols. Although we are all of course unique individuals, you will soon begin to notice there are some basic common traits among people with blue, brown, and mixed irides.

Eye colour does not follow the classical paths of inheritance. In fact, evidence suggests that as many as sixteen different genes could be responsible for eye colour in humans.[28]

Iridologists widely agree that there are **three** main constitutions determined by their colour.

They are:

- **Blue**—the lymphatic constitution
- **Brown**—the haematogenic constitution
- **Green/hazel**—the mixed biliary constitution

Each of the above categories also has a number of subtypes. However, it is not within the scope of this book to go into each one in depth. Should you be interested in delving further into the subject, a list of more detailed resources and reading materials can be found at the back of this book.

In general, we can make the observation that iris colour correlates to the general *function* of the body on a daily basis.

As I have already alluded, within the body of the iris, many different tones and shades will be apparent. This section focuses on the general iris colour, and the information this reveals at first glance. Further information on the subject of colours, shade, tones, markings and nuances will follow in the section covering the notion of diathesis (the iris overlay), where we will look in more depth at the nuances between other visible signs and markings.[29]

---

[28] Désirée White and Montserrat Rabago-Smith. "Genotype-phenotype associations and human eye colour" *Journal of Human Genetics* 56, (October 2011); 5–7 https://www.nature.com/articles/jhg2010126
[29] See Part 6: Patterns and markings. Pg 59.

The blue iris — the lymphatic constitution

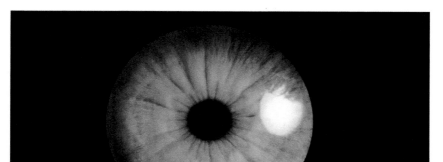

Historically, individuals with blue eyes tend to come from colder climates. Because of this, over many generations these individuals have developed a predisposition to hold onto body heat in order to stay warm. It's thought that this is the reason why blue-eyed individuals are generally more prone to inflammation and related conditions, such as arthritis or eczema.

Blue eyed individuals tend to be fair skinned with blonde or red hair. As the name suggests, lymphatic types are susceptible to *lymphatic congestion* and have a tendency towards a build-up of mucous and inflammation, which in turn can lead to an overactive immune system. People with blue eyes are generally more prone to coughs and colds, hay fever, catarrh, and allergies. They're also more likely to be challenged by auto-immune conditions.[30]

The pure blue iris has a tendency towards disorders of the upper respiratory tract. Blue eyed children often succumb to tonsilitis, ear infections, or skin eruptions. In early adulthood, inflammatory tendencies often manifest as asthma, wheezing or breathing problems, and

---

[30] Some practitioners have suggested that people with a pure lymphatic constitution have an abundance of white blood cells which contributes to their overactive immune system. Colton, *Iridology,* 49.

later on in life; arthritic joints, bladder infections, kidney stress, or more severe skin eruptions such as chronic psoriasis.

Key words to describe the blue iris type are:

• Inflammation
• Overactive immune system
• Skin problems
• Upper respiratory tract issues
• Heat in the mucous membranes

Some common health complaints associated with the lymphatic constitution are:

• Hay fever
• Asthma
• Eczema
• Allergies
• Auto-immunity
• Arthritis
• Recurrent urinary tract infections

Of course, not everyone will go on to develop these conditions, but the iris tells us that their inherited constitution means they are more *predisposed* to them.

Pure lymphatic types benefit from cleansing herbal teas which are supportive of the lymphatic system and kidneys; for example, Cleavers (*Galium aperine*), Dandelion leaf (*Taraxacum officinale*), Nettle (*Urtica dioica*), Celery seed (*Apium graveolens*), Echinacea (*Echinacea angustifolia/purpurea*) and simple lifestyle interventions, such as regular dry skin brushing. Avoiding mucous forming foods, such as dairy products, and eating an alkaline diet, avoiding refined sugar and processed meats, may also help to keep the constitution in balance.

The brown iris—the haematogenic constitution

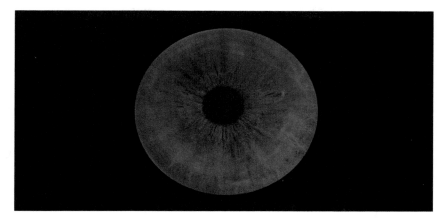

For the most part, people with brown eyes historically tend to originate from countries with hot climates. People with this type of constitution are prone to different sorts of health issues than those with blue or mixed irides.

The word "haem" comes from the Greek meaning "blood." As the name suggests, haematogenic types tend to be more predisposed to issues involving the blood, such as high cholesterol, anaemia, or problems with the circulatory system.

People with brown eyes are also more susceptible to health problems related to the liver and gallbladder (the organs that metabolise fat). This means they may also be more likely to gain weight or have difficulty extracting and storing certain minerals essential for maintaining good health. In adulthood, they may commonly experience problems such as varicose veins, arteriosclerosis, haemorrhoids, and endocrine disorders.

Energetically, people with pure brown eyes can be thought of as generally less "reactive" than the lymphatic type, and are more likely to complain of "cold" rather than hot, inflammatory conditions. Because they have more of a tendency towards accumulation, sluggishness and toxicity; lumps, bumps, and cysts are generally more prevalent among people with brown eyes. Their slower energetic profile means that although problems can take a longer time to manifest, they also take longer to resolve. This means that brown eyed individuals need to be extra careful not to ignore minor health issues, and address problems as they arise, in order to avoid developing more serious issues later on down the line.

Key words to describe the pure brown iris type are:

- Blood
- Metabolism
- Liver and gall bladder
- Nutrient absorption
- Lumps and bumps
- Stagnation

Some common health conditions associated with the brown iris type are:

- Cardiovascular disease
- Iron deficiency anaemia
- High blood pressure
- Diabetes
- Peripheral circulatory issues
- Gallstones

Herbs that nourish the blood and support the liver and circulatory system are helpful for this constitutional type. These include warming and moving herbs such as Ginger (*Zingiber officinale*), liver supportive bitters like Yellow-dock (*Rumex crispus*), or Barberry (*Berberis vulgaris*), circulatory supportive herbs such as Hawthorn berries (*Crateagus oxyanthus*), and vasodilatory herbs that help the blood to move freely, such as Lime blossom (*Tilia europea*).

People with brown eyes should try to include plenty of garlic, iron rich foods, and healthy fish oils into their diet. Warming spices, such as chillies and lemongrass, which move the blood, should also be regularly consumed.

Foods containing B vitamins help the absorption of iron, so should also be considered, as well as supplementing with trace minerals if there is a deficiency. Movement is absolutely key for this type. Cardiovascular exercise and exposure to sunlight is extremely beneficial. Exercising outdoors in the fresh air helps to re-oxygenate the blood, as well as provide vital vitamin D.

The mixed/green/hazel iris — the mixed biliary constitution

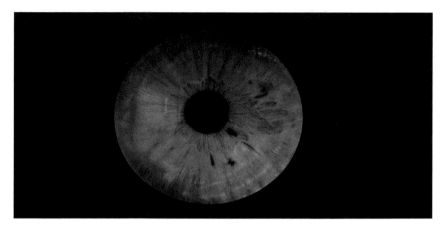

The mixed iris is usually observed as a blue iris with a brown over-lay, giving the eye the appearance of being green to golden in colour. The mixed iris can be very varied, displaying all manner of tones and shades from light green to very dark brown. In general, the pigment is usually darker in the centre of the iris, and fades away towards the edges, revealing the underlying colour. Sometimes crypts (holes in the iris structure) can also provide clues to the base colour underneath. When you're first starting out, the mixed constitution is generally the one that often proves most difficult to correctly identify.

There's some debate amongst iridologists as to whether or not this is indeed a third type or simply a mixture of the other two. If a person has more brown pigmentation in their iris, they'll naturally possess more tendencies of the haematogenic type. Lighter green eyes (a mixture of a blue underlay with yellow overlaid on top) indicates more of an influ-ence from lymphatic family members — hence a predisposition towards more lymphatic type health issues. Again, this highlights the impor-tance of diligent case taking to define which herbs and lifestyle inter-ventions are going to be most beneficial for each individual.

People with this constitution often experience the best and (there-fore by definition) the worst, of both iris types. This means they must walk a very fine line when it comes to looking after their health. When the mixed constitution is in balance they enjoy the best of both worlds, but they can quickly become out of sorts — particularly if they don't look after their delicate *digestive system*, which is a key theme for these individuals.

The full name for this iris is the "mixed biliary" constitution. This clue tells us that emphasis on the proper functioning of the liver, gall-bladder, and pancreas are crucial for this type.

Mixed constitutions have a tendency towards sluggish digestion, which is often due to a reduced supply of digestive enzymes. This leads to the improper breakdown of food particles, which can then enter the gut undigested. This commonly leads to a condition known as dysbiosis—an imbalance in the ratio of good and bad bacteria in the gut. In turn, this can cause metabolic deficiencies due to malabsorption of vital vitamins and minerals. It can also pre-dispose the individual to issues such as, candida overgrowth, and in rarer cases, a condition known as auto-brewer syndrome (a rarely diagnosed gut fermentation syndrome, whereby ingested carbohydrates are converted to alcohol by fungal overgrowth and a reduced population of healthy bacteria in the gastrointestinal tract.)

Key words to describe the mixed iris type are:

- Liver, gall bladder and pancreas
- Easily sent off balance
- Poor digestion and assimilation
- Compromised microbiome
- Lack of digestive enzymes

Common health conditions associated with the mixed iris type are:

- Candiasis and fungal infections (athlete's foot, thrush, dandruff)
- Irritable bowel syndrome
  Gas, bloating, indigestion

Herbs with bitter, sour taste profiles help stimulate the secretion of vital digestive enzymes often lacking with this type. The classic herbal formula Swedish bitters[31] is traditionally prescribed for aiding digestion, and the cooling formula is often prescribed for this constitution.

---

[31] Swedish bitters is a traditional herbal formula made popular by the Austrian herbalist Maria Treben.
Maria Treben, *Health Through God's Pharmacy*, 22nd Edition, (Steyer: Austria, Wilhelm Ennsthaler, 1994).

Apple cider vinegar is also known to help stimulate the flow of saliva and is a cheap and effective way to improve digestion. Taking a shot of apple cider vinegar before meals may also be helpful for supporting the digestion of the mixed biliary type.

Of course, liver supporting herbs should always be considered. This includes, Milk thistle (*Silybum marianum*), Rosemary (*Rosmarinus officinalis*), and Barberry (*Berberis vulgaris*) as well as carminative (wind relieving) herbs and spices generally added to food to aid digestion. These include Aniseed (*Pimpenella anisum*) Chamomile (*Matricaria recutita*), Fennel (*Foeniculum vulgare*) and Angelica (*Angelica archangelica*).

Eating slowly, avoiding heavy meals, or eating late at night is also sensible advice, as is reducing the consumption of alcohol and refined sugar (which compounds issues associated with candida overgrowth) and supporting the healthy balance of the microbiome with a good quality probiotic.

As in every case, the key is to always to tailor your advice to the individual. This means taking into account which constitution the client is leaning towards. If the client has a dark iris, you may need to tilt your advice towards the haematogenic type, whereas lighter irides may veer towards protocols best suited for lymphatic constitutions.

The central heterochromia

When first starting out, it's easy to trip up and make the mistake of confusing the true mixed biliary type with a lymphatic (blue) eye with a brown central heterochromia.

This central heterochromia is really just a concentrated area of colour or pigmentation which appears around the central portion of the iris.

The colour (which can be yellow, brown, or bright white) *only extends to the end of the digestive zone*[32] *but does not cover the entire iris.*

---

[32] This area of the chart covers both the stomach and intestines. See the section on charts for a more detailed explanation of the iris zones.

The picture below helps to illustrate this point.

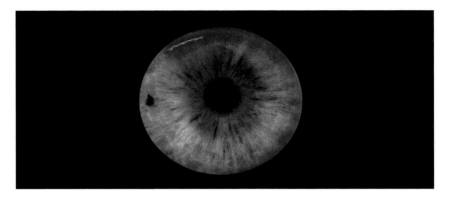

In this image, the main body of the iris is blue (lymphatic type,) but the central portion of the iris is clearly a different colour. The iris **as a whole** is not mixed. Essentially this is a blue iris with a brown colouration over the top of one clear area—the digestive zone, and is therefore **not** a classic mixed biliary type.

Telling the difference can feel difficult at first, but look closely and ascertain;

Does the overlaying colour extend throughout the entire iris, or just the central portion?

This central heterochromia is an indication that the person may have issues around the correct functioning of their digestive system. Depending on the colour and shape of the marking, there are a number of possible interpretations; from slow transit bowel to excess acid. Proper absorption of vitamins and minerals may be a concern, or there may be other issues around elimination, such as irritable bowel syndrome, chronic constipation, or even parasites.

Just like the classic mixed biliary types, focusing on the health of the liver, pancreas, and gallbladder is very important for these people. They may benefit from naturopathic gut rebalancing programs, and of course, proper attention to diet and what the person is eating (or not eating) on a daily basis, is always going to be an important consideration.

The colour of the heterochromia and the areas it covers will give you further clues as to what is going on in each individual case.[33]

---

[33] Refer to the information on colours in the later section on diathesis (page 59) to learn more about how to interpret this sign.

The stomach ring

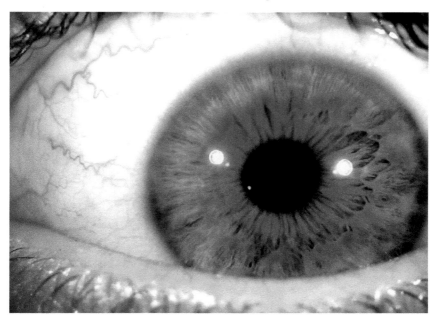

Another classic, commonly seen feature is the stomach ring. This is visible as a perfect circle next to the pupil and covering **only** the stomach zone (the area immediately surrounding the pupil), unlike the above example, it does not invade the intestinal zone. Just like the central heterochromia, the stomach ring can be white, yellow, or brown. Once again, it is the *colour* that is indicative of the sorts of problems that might be going on in that area. The photograph above clearly shows a perfect circle just around the pupil, but does not extend beyond and into the colon zone.

The difference between a stomach ring and a central heterochromia is that the stomach ring is **a clearly defined circle which only covers the stomach zone as opposed to the entire collarette,** (the area in between the pupil and the frilly rope like structure about a third of the way out towards the edge of the iris).

The photograph above is a clear example of a classic blue iris with a clearly defined brown stomach ring. Although we can also see more of the brown colouration further out towards the edges of the iris, the markings are clearly **outside the boundary of the autonomic nerve ring or collarette**.

Note the difference between this image and the one below which only has clear yellow markings in the bowel area (as opposed to the stomach area which is the area immediately surrounding the pupil.) This person is more likely to experience health issues with tone and motility in the lower intestine and colon, as opposed to digestive problems related to the stomach, (for example, excess acid or stomach ulcers.)

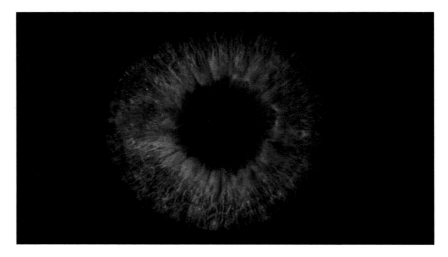

We'll talk more about the zones, the collarette, and the meaning of the different colours in the section relating to the iris map. For now, these photographs are merely aimed at helping you begin to discern the difference between a true mixed biliary type (in which the **entire iris** is a mixture of blue and brown pigment,) and a blue iris with coloured markings in clearly defined areas. It does take a little practice at first, but developing these observational skills really is key to determining a more bespoke healing protocol for your client.

Have a go at the following exercise which will help you gain more confidence telling the difference between the lymphatic, haematogenic and mixed biliary constitutions.

Exercise:
Make a mental note of the eye colour of the people you know. Practice becoming competent in identifying the three different colour constitutions. If you know the person well, try to correlate their health issues with their eye colour. Do they fit the picture? How typical are they of their constitutional type?

PART 5

Structure—your inherited disposition

What can be learned from the iris structure?

A person's constitution can be further defined by looking closely not just at the visible colour, but at the structure of the iris itself.

When you look closely at a person's eyes, you will notice that as well as the general eye colour, there are what appear to be fibres radiating out from the pupil towards the outer edge of the iris. These filaments are like little strands that have been unwound from a reel of thread, or a ball of wool. Sometimes they are very fine like the texture of silk, in other individuals they are much thicker, like rope or cables. These fibres may be zigzagged, close together or stretched apart like strings on a musical instrument. Sometimes there will be a tightly woven structure, in other individuals, the fibre structure may appear to be very open and loose.

These fibres represent the person's general structural type, and can be an indication of their natural resilience to illness and disease.

In reality, most people usually have a combination of one or more of the structural types. When you first start out, it can take a bit of practice to simplify what you're seeing in front of you. Features such as crypts, lacunae, and rarefaction (these are like little holes or threadbare patches in the iris—we'll talk more about this later,) can also complicate the picture. When you're starting out, it's a good idea to first look for a *general overall pattern*, before using an iridology chart to make notes of any denser areas or special features which may indicate weaknesses or issues in specific organs or body systems.

For now, try to focus an gaining an impression of the person's *general* disposition. For the purposes of simplicity, only the general characteristics of each of the types will be discussed.

Your inherited disposition

Different books use different terms to describe these structural patterns. Personally, I find it can be helpful to describe what you're looking at in terms of texture. Some books use the analogy of material to describe the texture, other books use wood grain for comparison. Using this kind of language helps to gain a feel for (and more easily classify) the general nature of the person's constitution inherited at birth.

A quick note before we begin:
It's important to remember that we all have our strengths and weaknesses. No one constitution is more desirable than another. Many times, it's our own personality and lifestyle choices that determine how robust or otherwise our constitution remains. Although the "strong" silk type (see below) is often considered to be the hardiest, if that person is burning the candle at both ends, eating junk food day and night, and generally going about their day pushing the limits and squandering their inherited predisposition, they're likely to end up being much worse off than a low resistance constitution who pays close attention to staying within their limits and actively works on looking after their health. The beauty of iridology lies in its capacity to help us learn ways to live in harmony with the physical, emotional and spiritual demeanour that nature has gifted us. Describing the iris in terms of texture and materials reminds us that we are all equally beautiful, we just exhibit different qualities, and therefore require different types of care.

Structural types

Silk

Key words: resilience, strength, tension, protection, resistance, adrenaline

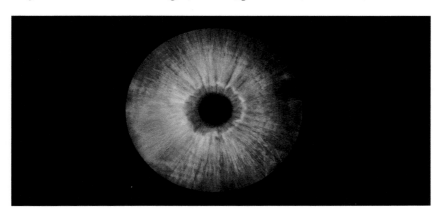

In older texts you may see this referred to as the "neurogenic" or *high resistance type*. These people have very tightly woven iris fibres which appear to be stretched taught like strings on a harp. In some people (particularly in brown iris types) the fibres can appear to be so close together they are almost invisible.

Silk types are often physically strong. Their ancestors were the boat builders of this world, able to withstand harsh physical activity and living conditions. They are the extreme sports enthusiasts who love to push themselves to the very limits of their capabilities. They are workaholics, perfectionists, high flying academics, and world leaders. They have chain mail armour defence against illness and disease, which at times makes them feel invincible. This is unfortunately their weak spot, often making them the masters of their own downfall.

The silk type has a tendency to believe they can go on forever. They push themselves beyond the normal limits of endurance, resulting in burnout, adrenal fatigue, and autoimmune conditions that stop them in their tracks. They are often not very good at opening up about their problems, preferring to "just get on with it" and "keep calm and carry on." The key feature for this iris type is to learn how to slow down and find time to rest and reset. Encouraging them to become more aware of their limitations is one thing, but getting them to actually do it is another. Silk types can be quite uptight when it comes to taking advice and being told what to do!

Health

The silk type is gifted with natural physical strength and an abundance of excess energy that simply has to be put to use. Their tendency to always be "on the go" puts their adrenal glands under enormous stress. In turn, this places a huge burden on the other organs in the HPTA (hypothalamus, pituitary gland, thyroid and adrenals) endocrine system, which can cause all manner of problems if left unattended, such as chronic fatigue or even ME.

Physically, silk types hold onto a lot of tension, which can manifest in many ways. Although their robust digestive system gives them a certain ability to eat what they like, their tightness and rigidity often results in constipation and congestion in the eliminatory channels. An overwrought nervous system predisposes silk children to develop poor bathroom habits (such as holding on until they are ready to go), which can continue into adulthood and become the norm. They may also eat "on the hop" meaning that they may convince themselves they have an excellent diet, but never take time to sit down and properly digest their meals. They often don't sit still long enough to properly chew their nutritious meals, and so can suffer with stomach acid, reflux, and even ulcers if they don't properly manage their stress and learn to slow down.

From an emotional perspective, they are often unable to "let go." This tension manifests as conditions such as migraines, high blood pressure, and muscular aches and pains. Their inability to switch off may mean they suffer from lack of sleep—the number one thing this type really needs in order to properly recharge.

Although physically strong, silk types often have the weakest nervous system. This is possibly due to the fact they are vulnerable to the influence of negative emotions, and try to avoid confronting them at all costs. Silk types often have small pupils, which, as we have seen, is a protective mechanism to keep things locked away inside. It's little wonder that practitioners of rayid iridology describe this as the "self protective" iris.

Supportive interventions

The silk type's obsessive need to expend energy leads either to physical exhaustion (or at the other end of the spectrum) pent up emotional problems such as anger, frustration, and even depression.

Their "just get on with it" attitude will make it hard for them to come to your office. Having a tendency to ignore ill health means that patterns can be well and truly established by the time they seek help. They view illness as weakness, forget to take medications, refuse advice and will sit in front of you and tell you with confidence they're perfectly happy and well. It's often a shock to them when they fall ill, and they can feel very frustrated that their body has "let them down". For this reason, encouraging them to spend some time journaling may be helpful. Silk types are much more likely to comply with your suggestions when they're able to reach their own conclusions, rather than simply being told what to do.

The key take-away for this type is that they need to become attuned to their limitations and slow down. As they are often unable to sit still, they should be encouraged to find ways to switch off by indulging in activities where they feel they are actually doing something, such as gardening or hiking.

As silk types already thrive on being in a high adrenaline state, using caffeine (and sometimes other substances) to keep pushing themselves further and beyond their limits should be strictly avoided.

Antispasmodic herbs such as Cramp bark (*Viburnum opulus*), Passionflower (*Passiflora incarnata*), and Chamomile (*Matricaria recutita*), along with nervine supportive herbs such as Skullcap (*Scutellaria lateriflora*) and Vervain (*Verbena officinalis*) may be helpful.

A deep tissue massage with appropriate, relaxing essential oils, as well as individually prescribed Bach flower remedies may help them examine their health issues from another angle and may also be good options.

Linen

Key words: balance, self-awareness, harmony

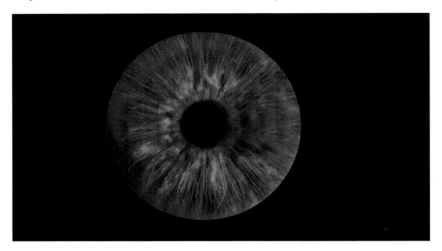

The most common iris type, the constitution of the linen person lies somewhere between the silk and hessian structural constitution. The iris fibres are not quite as fine or as close together as the silk type, nor are they as open or thick as the hessian eye. Most people fall into this middle area.

The linen iris has a less dense structural pattern than the silk type. In general, these types are somewhat more aware of their own physical boundaries. Because they don't go to extremes, they're generally able to live within their constitutional constraints, equally balancing work with rest.

Being somewhere in the middle, linen types are the sort of people who are happy to come to the practitioner's office whenever they're feeling below par. The linen individual is completely open to the idea that they can feel unwell even though they're not technically sick, and will seek advice about strategies to improve their wellbeing. Being self-aware means that linens are usually open to hearing advice about their health, and will generally listen to (and take on board) suggestions aimed at improving their wellbeing. They're the sort of person who would be delighted to walk out of your office with a "herbal tonic" and are usually compliant with both taking the medicine and implementing dietary changes and adopting better lifestyle choices in order to get results.

The biochemical function of linens often plays a greater role in their general health and wellbeing than their structure. When conducting an examination, pay attention to any special features such as crypts (obvious holes in the iris texture) markings, or deviations in the regular pattern, which will help you formulate an individual prescription.

In some books, you may also see this structural constitution referred to as the "cotton" iris type.

Supportive interventions

Although the linen type is often classed as "average", this doesn't mean that this constitution is undesirable. Not being at either extreme end of the spectrum is a definite advantage. In short, it means that with reasonable care and attention to lifestyle and diet, balance is much more easily achieved.

Supportive interventions should focus on the iris colour and constitutional type, as well as addressing specific health concerns. Creating an herbal tea blend they can sip throughout the day may also be a good option, as this type of client is much more likely to want to take an active role in improving their general wellbeing.

Hessian

Key words: structural weakness, metabolic accumulation, mineral deficiency, joints, bone health, personal boundaries, creativity, unpredictable energy patterns

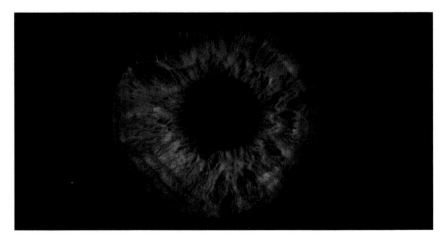

In this type, the iris fibres have the appearance of a more open, coarse weave. There are often twists, kinks, and even knotting of the fibres, which can in places be of irregular thickness. The hessian structure is

much more open than the silk and linen type, and far less uniform. In this respect, they can be considered to be more sensitive to outside stimuli such as light, noise, people and even the weather. This sensitivity to stimuli means they are often inventors, writers and dreamers, and thrive when they're able to express themselves creatively.

From a personality perspective, hessian types are social creatures. In the workplace, they make good team players, preferring to work in groups where tasks can be shared. Unlike the silk type they are fully aware of their limitations and do not like to push themselves beyond their physical capacities.

Health

Hessian types have less physical stamina than some of the other structural dispositions. They know when they need to take rest and relaxation (and are more than happy to do it.) Hessian types are easily fatigued; so adequate rest and sleep must be a priority, particularly after an illness where the recuperation period may be longer than other, more robust constitutions.

Hessian types should, however, be mindful of taking extra care of their musculoskeletal system. They cannot physically abuse their bodies without suffering the consequences, which manifest as chronic aches and pains, prolapses, and slow healing of injuries. They may also be prone to structural weaknesses in the lower back, and spinal misalignments. They should avoid sitting at desks for long periods of time, or engaging in repetitive activities that place a burden on the same muscles or joints.

Being more aware of their constitution, these types do not often suffer with burnout. On the other hand, their relaxed attitude to life sometimes means they don't take as much care as they could of their diet or physical wellbeing. Eating well is important if the hessian type wants to avoid storing up long-term problems, as poor metabolism of minerals is likely to exacerbate their predisposition towards structural weakness.

Special attention should also be paid to avoiding the build up of metabolic waste in the kidneys and muscle fibres, another condition to which they are prone.

Supportive interventions

The Hessian type has a tendency to become easily depleted, therefore emphasis should firmly be placed on using their energy reserves wisely. They would benefit from engaging in weight-bearing activities, such as kettle bells, and taking mineral rich nutritional supplements, such as seaweeds and spirulina.

Adaptogenic herbs for stamina may be helpful. This includes herbs such as Eleuthero (*Eleutherococcus senticosus*), and Rhodiola (*Rhodiola rosea*). Herbs that support the adrenal glands, such as Liquorice (*Glycyrrhiza glabra*) and Rehmannia (*Rehmannia glutinosa*), may also be helpful.

Hessian types should avoid stimulants including caffeine, refined sugar, and alcohol. Regular visits to the chiropractor to keep on top of musculoskeletal health will also be beneficial. Sleep hygiene and the creation of a regular nighttime routine should also be encouraged.

Net

Key words: connective tissue, receptive, self-awareness, instinctive, adaptive sensitivity

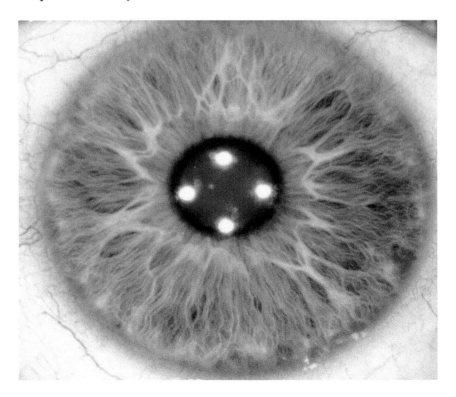

The net iris is the opposite of the tightly woven, taught, fine fibres seen in the silk type. The typical pattern is reminiscent of one of those trendy shopping bags made from string. The iris often has the appearance of whitish, loose fibres and is more commonly seen in people with blue eyes; in fact, I have yet to meet a haematogenic person displaying this structural type.

The fibres in the net iris are far less numerous than the other structural types. As such, you'll often see it referred to as the "low density" iris. Like a fisherman's net, this iris pattern is made up of an interwoven mesh of many holes. However, this doesn't necessarily equate to weakness. Think of the weight that can be hauled in a trawler net, or the pliable spider's web that withstands the strongest winds. Nets can be as strong as steel cables, but one weak chink can compromise the entire structure. This is how it is with the net individual. The open structure of the iris implies a less robust disposition, yet this sensitivity could be in fact be considered a great advantage.

The net person is unpredictable in their strength. One moment they are exhausted, the next they get a second wind are full of vim. Unlike silk types who have a tendency to push themselves to the very brink of their limits, net people have an amazing capacity to self-regulate, and so rarely reach a point where they run out of reserves. They heed the messages their bodies send them, and take precautions to manage their health before illness takes hold.

Because of the lack of fibre density, the eye is able to take in more light. In theory it could be argued that this means nerve endings are more easily stimulated making the net individual much more sensitive than other types. In rayid iridology, these are the people who are able to see more clearly beyond the everyday, and perhaps even have psychic tendencies.

Health

Net types are prone to connective tissue weakness. They're susceptible to prolapses, joint issues, carpal tunnel syndrome, organ displacement, arthritis, haemorrhoids, and suchlike. Some net individuals have hypermobility of joints. These are the people who perform amazing contortion acts, or the lithe magician's assistant able to bend into unnatural positions at will. Net types may have issues with dislocating limbs or suffer with cartilage damage, and so taking care of the musculoskeletal system is of paramount importance.

Physiologically, there may be difficulty transporting oxygen and nutrients to where they're needed, and poor lymphatic drainage (as evident in the blue-eyed lymphatic type) increases the likelihood of toxicity building up in the tissues.

Interestingly, most of the net individuals I've met seem to be rather placid people who have the enviable ability to appear totally unphased by stress. Perhaps being aware of their limits allows them the luxury of being able to ignore anything which might threaten to overload them— a natural defense mechanism designed to protect their finite energy reserves. However, whenever pain is involved, this is a very different story. Net types have a very low pain threshold (both emotional and physical), which can make them feel quite vulnerable. It can take them quite a long time to recover from injuries or emotional shocks, and they often need a lot of sleep and rest to recover.

Supportive interventions

In complete contrast to the silk type, the net individual has very low resistance. If a net type is feeling overstretched (energy management is a common reason for finding themselves in your office), they can have a tendency to feel spaced out. Net types are prone to using diversion or avoidance techniques to disassociate from their stressful situation. Energy conservation means they may not have the reserves to take on new health regime and so herbs and therapeutic interventions will need to be supportive and require less effort on their part if the person is going to comply.

The net type should avoid strenuous exercise, which can rapidly deplete their reserves. If exercise is required, (for example, to help build stamina or strength), then low impact options such as Pilates or swimming are best.

This structural disposition is most commonly found among blue iris types and so attention must also be paid to improving drainage through the kidneys and proper transportation of nutrients and oxygen around the body.

Carefully chosen, stamina building herbs may be helpful. Consider gentle adaptogens, such as Astragalus (*Astragalus membranaceus*),

Wild Oats (*Avena sativa*), and Ashwagandha (*Withania somnifera*). Albizia (*Albizia julibrissin*) is indicated in cases where the person is recovering from a physical or emotional injury. They may also benefit from energetic medicines such as homeopathic preparations and Bach flower remedies.

Mixed structures

Some irides appear to have a mixture of open and closed textures, which when starting out, can make it difficult to know what structural type a person fits into. The following structural types are common patterns, which can have their own distinct set of health issues and traits. Again, with practice, you will soon begin to learn how to differentiate between the different structural patterns you are seeing.

The daisy iris (poly-glandular type)

Key words: hormones, emotions, sugar cravings, fertility issues, candida

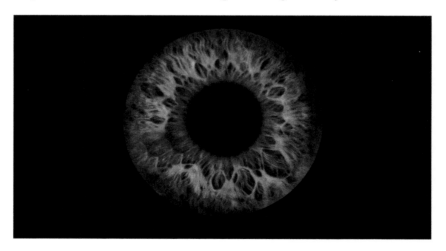

Polyglandular people are often noted for their distinctive iris pattern which has the appearance of "daisy-like" flower petals (which are really teardrop-shaped holes or crypts) *outside* the collarette. There must be

three or more petals present for the person to be classified as a poly-glandular type.

Health

People with this constitutional type are predisposed to problems associated with the endocrine system, which in many cases (most notably when combined with a mixed iris) are usually aggravated by improper digestive function.

Polyglandular types tend to have lowered function of the adrenal, thyroid, and pituitary gland, and so often suffer with issues such as irregular periods, lethargy, and unexplained weight gain. Polycystic ovarian syndrome, metabolic disorders, and even infertility are common in people with this type of iris. Type II diabetes may also manifest later on in life, due to a tendency towards adrenal fatigue, and pancreatic burnout, which further reduces their ability to regulate their blood sugar.

Supportive interventions

As well as prescribing herbs that support the endocrine system, it's paramount to offer sensible digestive support. Polyglandular types should avoid eating a diet high in carbs and refined sugar, and avoid consuming too much alcohol. They need to take regular gentle exercise to help metabolise excess hormones, but avoid high impact physical activities which place additional stress on the adrenal glands.

Herbs which help to control blood sugar such as Burdock (*Arcticum lappa*), Barberry (*Berberis vulgaris*), and Gymnema (*Gymnema sylvestris*), should be considered, as well as Swedish bitters, which is a popular over-the-counter pre-blended mix of digestive supportive herbs to help increase enzymes for the proper breakdown and elimination of food.

The gastric iris

Key words: gut health, candida, dysbiosis, rigidity, instincts, constipation

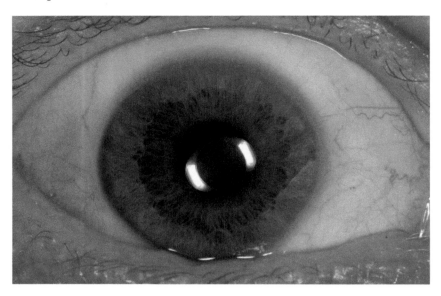

At first glance, it's easy to confuse the gastric iris with the daisy type. However, the main difference between the two is that the gastric iris also has multiple visible lacunae (large open or closed holes in the iris structure) *inside* the collarette. This characteristic means that the collarette will often appear to be as large (if not larger) than the space outside of it. The lacunae will often have what appears to be even smaller holes (crypts) within them. The iris will, therefore, appear to have two distinct zones; the looser texture filled area with gaps and holes within the collarette, and the rest of the eye, appearing robust and "silk" like.

Health

The main concerns for people who display this type of constitution tend to focus around digestion. This includes complaints such as excess stomach acid, bloating, diverticulitis, dysbiosis, and candiasis (disruption of the delicate balance of bacteria within the gut microbiome which leads to the overgrowth of *candida albicans*.) They may suffer with thrush, fungal infections and issues related to impaired elimination.

The majority of gastric types experience issues with constipation and the breaking down of food, which may take a longer time to pass through the bowel. Like the silk type, the gastric type has a tendency to hold on to their emotions and often find it difficult to let go of hurtful remarks and unresolved arguments. They can be creatures of habit, which can be helpful if they are working on creating a positive health plan, but detrimental if they are too rigid in their ideas and set in their ways to take advice.

On a positive note, they often act on their gut instincts and can be very self aware, relying on their own interpretation of events instead of looking outside of themselves for explanations.

Supportive interventions

Herbs and foods that focus on supporting bowel motility and increasing peristalsis are going to be very beneficial for the gastric constitution. Consider things like Dandelion root, Aloe Vera juice, and Psyllium husks. In stubborn cases the uses of stronger purgative herbs, such as Yellow Dock (*Rumex crispus*) or Black walnut shells (*Juglans nigra*) may be helpful, as well as undertaking a tailored gut rebalancing programme to re-establish healthy microbiota.

It is noteworthy to mention that people with this type of constitution are prone to parasites and may benefit from undertaking a regular bowel cleansing programme. In this instance consider antiparasitic herbs such as Wormwood (*Artemisia absinthium*) or Papaya enzymes.

Papaya fruit (*Carica papaya*) is particularly useful when working with children who cannot tolerate such strong doses of anthelmintic preparations. Papaya enzymes can be bought quite cheaply online and taken in small doses at regular intervals can serve as a useful preventative measure.

Following an anti-candida programme to rebalance the gut microbiome makes it harder for parasites to make themselves at home. Eliminating sugar and reducing the amount of refined carbohydrates in the diet alongside herbs such as Echinacea (*Echinacea* spp.) and other anticandidal herbs may be of help.

If you're working with a person with a gastric constitution, ask them about the amount of fibre they consume and how often they visit the bathroom for a bowel motion. Transit time can easily be established by performing a simple beetroot test before and after treatment to assess how well the suggested interventions are working.[34] Taking a short walk after mealtimes, avoiding eating late at night, and not drinking cold drinks at the same time as eating meals is going to be very helpful for this type.

---

[34] Food is not meant to hang around in the gut longer than twenty-four hours. A bowel transit time test measures how long it takes for food to travel through your digestive system. Eating a beetroot and monitoring how long it takes for the stool to appear red can give you an idea of how slowly (or quickly) food is passing through the gastrointestinal tract.

PART 6

Patterns and markings

Diathesis: the iris overlay

As you become more familiar with looking at the iris, you'll begin to notice that the eyes have many subtle tones and shades of colour. In addition to the genetically inherited base colour of the iris, it's also possible to see other hues and patterns in the eyes which have a wide variety of meanings. These patches, spots clouds, streaks and other markings are known as the iris "diathesis" or overlay, and can be an indication that certain organs or systems are not functioning quite as well as they could be. In medical terms *dyscrasia* means "disturbance through toxic overload of the blood, lymph, or connective tissue."

Some iridologists believe that colourations and markings appear due to inorganic substances settling in the tissues—in short, they are a sign of toxic accumulations and environmental pollutants. As very few people are in the habit of regularly taking photographs of their eyes right from the point of birth, it is unclear if these colours and markings change as we progress through life.[35]

Until there is hard evidence to suggest otherwise (and what a brilliant project this would be), it is my own personal belief that if subtle changes do take place, then the process is so slow and minute that it would be very difficult indeed to document. However, I would be delighted to be proven wrong.

This does put into question the many claims found on the internet that extreme detoxification can change the colour of a person's eyes. Although I do believe that tissue cleansing certainly brightens a person's features, it is hardly likely to make such a dramatic change in the appearance of the iris. In my opinion, these sorts of claims do nothing to promote the serious study of iridology, and should quite rightly be viewed with scepticism.

Personally, I like the description given by my US colleague Betty Sue O'Brian in her classic iridology textbook[36] that "pigmentation is nature's way of covering up and protecting a weaker area." Just as the pigment in our skin darkens with exposure to the sun, perhaps so does a similar process occur in the iris to protect the respective reflex zones.

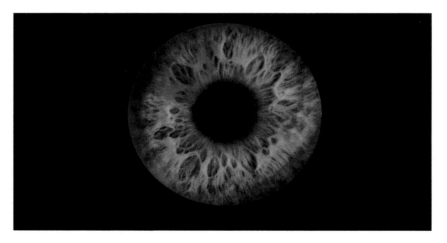

---

[35] In the process of writing this book, I compared photographs of my own irides taken as a twenty-three-year-old student, with a current photograph taken just last month. Placed side by side, I was unable to distinguish any significant differences between the two. This is despite the fact I have undoubtedly been exposed to any number of environmental toxins since then.

[36] Betty S. O'Brian, *The Core Curriculum Iris Analysis Manual,* 1st Revision (USA: Self-Published, 2016).

As we've already seen, the central heterochromia is a clear example of an *overlay*. When looking at different colours present in the iris, it is always handy to compare any visible markings to the general colour of the rest of the iris.

For example:

- A white foggy haze in the zone corresponding to the lung area[37] of an otherwise perfectly clear brown iris could be an indication of catarrh and a build-up of mucous in this organ.
- Brown colouration in the stomach area of a pale blue iris could be an indication of a slow transit bowel.

Although you will find many different hues and tones in the eye, the following chart will help to serve as a simple reference guide if you're just starting out.

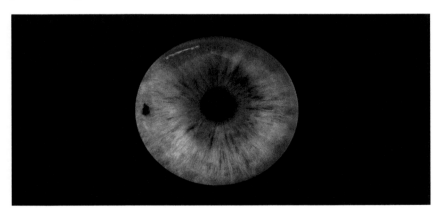

As well as a central heterochromia, there is a clear dark spot at 9 o'clock[38] (on the left of the image) which correlates on the charts to the lung area. As this is a clear and obvious marking, it would be prudent to ask about the client's respiratory health or any problems that may have been inherited as a past "miasm."

---

[37] Refer to the charts in Part 7—Finding your way around the iris. See Pg 68—The Iris "Clock."

[38] Refer to the charts in Part 7: Finding your way around the iris on Pg 67.

Colours and what they mean

When looking at the iris, bear in mind that colour demotes **bodily functions.**

White: This can indicate inflammation, irritation, or over-acidity of the tissues. It's most often seen in the blue iris type. As we've already seen over-activity is a common theme with the lymphatic individual. The brighter the colour, the more reactive a person tends to be.

When white is seen in the stomach zone[39] it may be a sign of excess stomach acid. Ask the person about their diet. Do they consume a lot of acid forming foods such as red meat, refined sugar, and dairy? Do they suffer with heartburn or indigestion?

White iris fibres are an indication of irritation, pain, discharge, and heat. It may be a sign that nervous energy is being used up at a rapid rate, or the person has a general tendency towards inflammatory processes. Ask them about issues such as gout, recurrent urinary tract infections, joint pain, and conditions ending in "itis" (arthritis, gastritis etc.)

Yellow: From my own personal experience, yellow often indicates a "liverish" constitution. It shows heat in the body which may be caused by impaired function of an organ, or conditions that have been present for long periods of time. In some cases, it may be an indication of poor fat metabolism. This is particularly the case if small yellow lumps are visible in the sclera. In medical terms this is known as a *pinguecula.* These bumps or growths may contain a combination of protein, fat, or calcium, or a combination of all three and are an indication that the body is not metabolising well.

In some cases, yellow markings in the iris can also be a sign that the kidneys are not excreting waste as well as they could. As we have already seen, a completely yellow sclera (the white part of the eye) should always be treated as a red flag. This is usually an indication of a serious health condition (for example, hepatitis) and is not a job for the iridologist.

Orange: This is often a sign that the person does not metabolise carbohydrates very well. There may be an inherited weakness in the pancreas and liver. Blood sugar issues may be a concern.

---

[39] Ibid.

Brown: In general, brown patches indicate a slowing down of energy, or hypo-function of the corresponding organs. As we have already seen, brown markings are commonly noted in the digestive zone, which is often affected by slow transit. Brown markings usually indicate chronic conditions or weaknesses inherited from previous generations. In this case, providing you take measures to avoid aggravating the issue, it may never present as a problem.

Black: Black is an indicator of long standing, chronic, or hereditary conditions.

Fog, clouds, and whisps: Cloudiness indicates an accumulation of metabolic acid waste which has built up in the tissues. It may show a tendency towards acidic conditions such as arthritis and gout. Avoiding acidic foods such as pork and coffee is advised. The person may benefit from a deep tissue cleansing programme, or drinking purifying juices made from celery and lemon. Cleansing herbs such as Celery (*Apium graviolens*), Nettle (*Urtica dioica*), and Dandelion (*Taraxacum officinale*) to support the liver and kidneys are also helpful.

When taking a case, always be sure to make a note of the size and location of any markings (along with their shape and colour) to inform your questioning and help you build up a more accurate picture of what's going on inside the body.

Lacunae, Crypts, and Rarefication

These signs are essentially *the opposite* of a pigmentation spot where instead of excess, a deficiency or weakness in the respective organ is implied.

Lacuna: These are gaps of various shapes and sizes, which are mostly enclosed (sometimes they are open), permanent, genetic markings in which the fibres are missing. They can come in a wide variety of shapes including leaf, rugby ball, capsule, peanut, or torpedo. As the terminology often varies in different texts, it's fun to read the different descriptions that are given to these features.[40]

---

[40] An excellent description of the various types of lacunae can be found in Chapter 7 of O'Brian, *Core Curriculum*, 62–67.

When three or more closed lacunae are seen in either the polyglandular or the gastric eye, the significance of each lacuna is not as important as the overall constitutional picture.

Crypt: These are very dark, deep, small lacunae that often penetrate through many layers. They are usually diamond shaped and can be found in any location of the iris.

Rarefication: An area in the iris in which the fibres appear to be less dense or even missing. This is a sign of general weakness in that area, for which long-term, supportive measures are usually required.

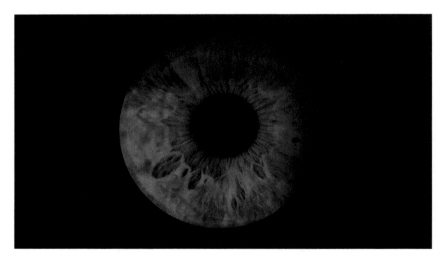

In the image above, large lacunae are visible at 7 and 8 o'clock, along with a dark pigmentation spot at 3 o'clock.

PART 7

Finding your way around the iris: how to use an iridology chart

Choosing your chart

The idea that one part of the body contains clues about the whole is not unique to iridology. Reflexologists, acupuncturists, people who practice palmistry, and Chinese face readers have all, since antiquity, developed their own charts to illustrate this concept.

Over the course of time, iridology has been studied and practiced throughout the world with many different iridology charts being developed independently of one another. Most agree on the basic positions with the main difference being in the amount of detail shown. One of the most influential charts was designed by Bernard Jensen, and many modern charts are based on his original drawings.[41]

As part of his PhD, Dr. Emil Bewö-Lundblad from Sweden sought to answer the question: *Does Iridology Have a Unified Map?* He presented

---

[41] Although there are many iris maps available, my advice to beginners is always to use the most updated version possible, and stick to it. Details of where to purchase charts can be found in the reference section.

his findings at the 21st Annual Iridology Symposium of the Guild of Naturopathic Iridologists in October 2018 in London.[42]

He selected nine individual iridology charts used in different parts of the world. The nine comparison charts were laid on top of each other as individual layers. At the end of his experiment, all of the charts used to make his comparisons were combined into the new *MICUC—Master Iridology Combined Unique Chart*.

In general, the original charts showed many similarities, but there were some exceptions that could not be explained without further studies. This clearly demonstrates that iridology is a complex science that gives rise to many varying interpretations. As such, there is no one standard chart that accurately represents the entire individual human body. The conclusion was reached that iridology is a complex subject which is open to a variety of different interpretations. There is therefore a need for standardisation to be acknowledged as an approved method of analysis.

As with reflexology and acupuncture charts, there are many different options available on the market.

Before making any decisions about which one is going to feel right for you, my suggestion would be to order a few different charts and then choose one that you are drawn to working most with. "Pick and stick" is really the best option. By sticking with one chart rather than trying to constantly cross reference, you will gain confidence much more quickly. You don't need to memorise everything—remember a chart can only provide so much information. It's the subtle clues that cannot be represented on a chart that are often some of the most important. Things like pupil size, a disturbance in shen, and unusual markings, can only be interpreted by a competent practitioner. It takes time and practice to develop this subtle skill.

Using the chart in practice

The general logic behind the iris chart is simple.

Imagine an apple core going right through the top of your head and piercing all the way through the central portion of your body.

---

[42] Helena Pike, "Iridology—One science or many?", The Guild of Naturopathic Iridologists International. December 2, 2018. https://www.gni-international.org/iridology-one-science-or-many-new-research/.

The central part of the chart (the area around the pupil) relates to the entire gastrointestinal tract, or as I like to think of it—the inner "pipe" of the body. The chart then works outwards, including all the major organs, and culminating in the outside ring of the chart which marks the boundary of where you end, and the outside world begins (your skin).

The top portion of the chart refers to the upper section of the body, and the bottom, well … to the bottom! Equally, the left side of the chart corresponds to the left-hand side of the body, and the right, to the right.

One of the most important things to remember is that as iridology charts are mostly used by practitioners to look into other people's eyes (who will always be facing them) the charts are printed "back to front." When you look at a chart, you'll notice a letter "R" to represent the right eye and a letter "L" to represent the left.

CHART OF IRIS TOPOGRAPHY
The College of Holistic Iridology

Developed by Peter Jackson-Main MSc FAMH FGNI
Copyright 2019

Note: The chart I personally prefer to work with is the one designed by my tutor Peter Jackson-Main and was the one I became familiar with as a student. I like the fact it isn't too over complicated, yet still provides enough detail to enable a precise reading. It's perfect for the beginner who is learning to find their way around. Information about where to purchase charts can be found in the reference section at the end of the book.

The iris zones

The next important thing to note is that the chart is roughly divided into zones. These zones radiate outwards from the centre, and there are six of them:

- The pupil
- The stomach and intestines zone
- The collarette or autonomic nerve wreath
- The assimilation zone
- The elimination zone—skin, lymph, skeletal structure.
- The outer border of the iris—the non-physical, aura which is the ethereal "envelope" of your physical body.

The iris "clock"

Some charts also have numbers around the outside edge, a little bit like a clock face. These numbers are represented by "minutes," with number 12 or a zero at the top. This is a handy way to record what you are seeing in your notes, as well as having the advantage of being easily understood by any other practitioners the client may be working with.

You can use this "minute system" to record the location of any significant markings. An example of this might be dark pigmentation at thirty minutes, or a cigar shaped lacuna at five o'clock.

The zones, along with the numbers on the outer edge of the chart, will help you learn how to locate important markings in the iris and navigate your way around it.

The collarette (or autonomic nerve wreath)

Before you begin to use any chart, it helps to be able to identify specific parts of the iris. I like to think of these as "landmarks" to help you find your way around more easily. One of the most important features you need to be aware of in order to locate important areas of the map is a feature often called the collarette or the autonomic nerve wreath.[43]

It's a helpful landmark because everybody has one, and it's very easy to locate.

---

[43] We've already briefly discussed this important iris feature in the section on the central heterochromia on Pg 39, and will discuss it again in more detail in the section on common collarette signs on Pg 77.

The collarette is a roughly circular structure of specialised muscle tissue that is controlled by the autonomic nervous system. It's located around the pupil (about a third of the way out towards the edge of the iris) and looks a little bit like a frilly circle. You'll notice it because it will appear to be slightly raised up from the rest of the iris. Its appearance varies greatly between individuals. In some people it can be virtually invisible, while in others it may appear to be very prominent and jagged, like the sides of a mountain range. In some people it forms a tight circle around the pupil, while in others it may appear to reach out all the way to the edge of the iris. As we've seen in our discussion about the central heterochromia, it is sometimes marked by a distinctly different colour.

As the name suggests, the autonomic nerve wreath provides us with a lot of information about the state of a person's nervous system, but it also marks the boundary between the digestive organs and the rest of the body. The stomach, and small and large intestines are all located inside the collarette.

More specific examples of the different collarette types can be found in the section on special signs.[44]

Exercise: studying your own eyes

Now that you've had a chance to familiarise yourself with the chart, it's time to put all you've learned into practice and make a study of your own eyes.

Remember the chart is designed to look at the person facing you, so before you begin, you are going to need to convert it for looking at yourself.

To make a reverse iridology chart for self-analysis, simply place an "R" over the "L" on the original chart and an "L" over the "R" so that the right eye becomes the left, and the left eye becomes the right.

Now you have your chart set, you can begin to take a deeper look at the position of any interesting markers in your iris. Make notes about your observations, remembering to go through your checklist and include the colour, structure, and any obvious markings you observe.

How closely does your study match your personal constitution and current health concerns?

---

[44] See Pg 71.

PART 8

Special signs

Contraction furrows

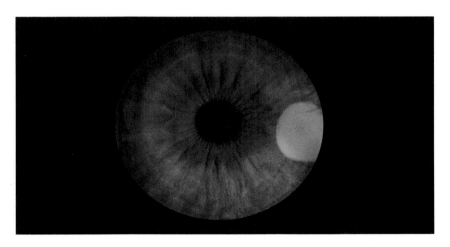

Extending around the iris like little waves rippling across a stream, contraction or "stair step" furrows can be partial or entire, and lie at various "depths." Many iridologists refer to these as "nerve rings." They're

71

often seen in conjunction with radial furrows (see below) in people who have a nervous disposition, hold tension in the musculoskeletal system, or have a tendency to internalise their stress. Breaks in the rings may indicate areas where stress is causing a particular problem.

These common markings are often more visible in silk and linen type individuals who have a particular tendency to keep their emotions under control rather than find useful ways to release any pent-up stress and frustration.

People with contraction furrows may benefit from supplementing with calcium and magnesium—the main minerals for supporting the nervous system. Helpful herbs may also include Cramp Bark (*Viburnum opulus*), Passionflower (*Passiflora incarnata*), Lemon Balm (*Melissa officinalis*), and Chamomile (*Matricaria recutita*).

Radial furrows (or "wagon wheel" spokes)

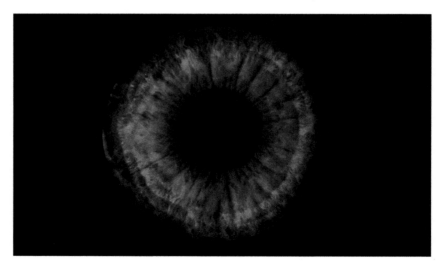

These markings are again commonly seen in people who suffer with anxiety and nervous tension. As the name suggests, these deep furrows appear to look like little wagon wheel spokes, and extend from the pupil or collarette, right up to the iris edge. If visible in the iris, it's worthwhile probing deeper with your questioning around bowel and digestive health, as well as inquiring about the person's stress levels and propensity to worry. In some cases, they are indicative of potential "leakage" from a congested bowel, causing issues such as headaches (particularly if terminating in the head area) or acid build up in the organs of elimination, such as the skin and kidneys.

People displaying radial furrows and contraction rings usually benefit from therapies such as massage, Bowen therapy, or acupuncture. Digestive, calming herbal teas which support both the digestive and nervous system (such as Chamomile or Lime blossom) are also a nice adjunct to a formula. Pulse point roller balls containing soothing essential oils like Lavender or Rose geranium to support an overwrought nervous system may also be a helpful suggestion.

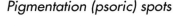

Pigmentation (psoric) spots

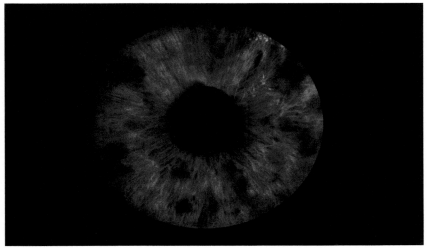

These are brown, red, or black pigmentation spots that form a scattered pattern. They resemble little freckles floating in between the iris and the clear corneal layer, and may in fact have a similar purpose.

The location of these spots is significant, and the organs affected can be located using an iridology chart. However, as with the polyglandular and gastric iris types who have many visible crypts, when the pattern of pigmentation is numerous, it is much more helpful to pay attention to the generalised picture rather than focus attention on each and every spot.

Pigmentation generally signifies an excess, or an accumulation of waste in the corresponding areas of the body. It can also imply a blockage of energy such as in the case of gallstones. People who practice emotional iridology have a more metaphysical view of this picture. They believe that the purpose of the spots is to protect a certain area of vulnerability, or in fact, are obscuring a particular area which prevents the person from "seeing clearly". In Chinese medicine, the organs have other functions that also relate to the emotions—e.g. the liver is associated with anger—so, where there is a spot in the iris covering a particular organ, it may be a clue that the person has a karmic lesson to learn or an obstacle to overcome, which must be dealt with before any healing can take place.[45]

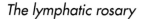

The lymphatic rosary

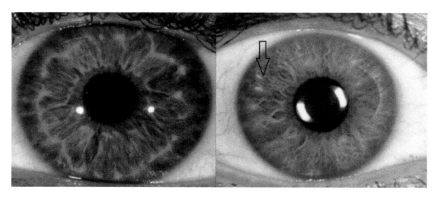

This is a ring of distinct spots around the edge of the iris which often appear in pairs. These spots are sometimes referred to as "tophi" and as already discussed; the sign is far more common in blue-eyed people. As in this image, the spots can sometimes appear to be joined up.

White spots signify hyper-reactivity and a potentially overactive immune system. There is congestion in the lymphatic channels and there may be a predisposition towards swollen glands, hay fever or swollen lymph nodes in the neck, armpits, and groin. Occasionally the spots are yellow, which may indicate a build-up of uric acid in the tissues, pre-disposing the person to gout. I have never personally seen brown lymphatic rosary spots visible in an iris.

---

[45] Dorothy Hall, *Iridology*, (London: Piatkus, 1994), 123.

Supportive interventions

Follow the advice for the lymphatic constitution.

Cholesterol rings

Also referred to as sodium or lipemic rings, this well-recognised iris sign looks like a whitish arc or thick opaque ring around the outer edge of the iris.[46] It is seen in all eye colours and iris types, although it is most common among people with brown eyes due to their constitutional tendency towards poor metabolism of fat.

The cholesterol ring is a genetic sign that develops in individuals aged forty and upwards, and is visible in people who have a tendency towards atherosclerosis and high cholesterol. It is an indicator of potential issues with circulation and blood pressure, as well as other cardiovascular issues. About 50% of people with this sign will go on to develop high cholesterol.

Individuals who display this sign often have liver imbalances, which cause improper metabolism of glucose and fat. In these cases, a yellowish deposit resembling a fatty deposit may also be found in the white of the eye. This sign further confirms the body's ability to break down fat from the diet.

When the ring is only partial and viewed at the top of the iris, it is referred to as the *arcus senilis* (the arc of old age). In this case, it may be an indicator of poor circulation to the head and brain. The ring is quite common among the elderly.

Practitioners of Rayid term this sign the "ring of determination", as it is often observed in individuals who have fixed patterns of belief and are somewhat set in their ways.

If a client appears in your office with this sign, ask them questions such as:

- Do they have cold hands and feet?
- Do they ever experience episodes of dizziness or palpitations?
- How is their memory?
- Do they have any varicose veins?
- Do they eat a healthy diet?

---

[46] See Pg 2.

Ask them about their family history and any other medications they may be taking, but most importantly, impress on them the importance of making an appointment with their GP to have their cholesterol checked.

Herbs to consider are Hawthorn (*Crateagus monogyna*), Linden (*Tilia europea*), and Motherwort (*Leonorus cardiaca*). The person should be encouraged to add chillies, garlic, and warming spices like ginger and galangal to food.

The scurf rim

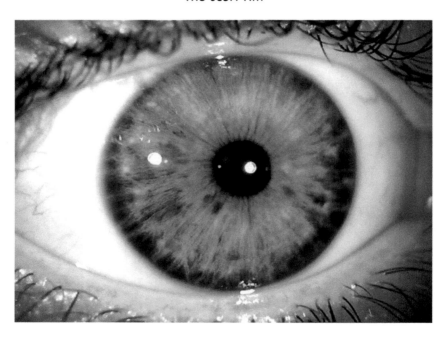

The scurf rim is a very dark area located at the outer edge of the iris. Unlike the cholesterol ring, it is dark in colour and almost appears to look like there's a part of the iris "missing." This is the zone of elimination and it provides us with a great deal of information in regards to the functioning of the skin.[47]

---

[47] Not to be confused with the cholesterol ring (which is always white or foggy) or the venous or anemic ring (which appears to be whitish blue).

People with this sign are less able to handle the build-up of metabolic waste products produced by the body. Poor elimination leads to a build-up of toxins and waste products that need to be mobilised or will potentially lead to conditions such as acne or eczema. It can also lead to pent up anguish and frustration if the person is unable to release their emotions or express themselves in a healthy way.

Wherever a scurf rim is seen, it's important to improve the function of all the organs of elimination—the liver, bowels, and kidneys. These people should also avoid using heavy make-up or cleansing products that may block the pores, and will usually benefit from a gentle naturopathic cleansing programme.

Supportive interventions

People who display a prominent scurf rim would benefit from regular use of a sauna or dry skin brushing. This popular herbal spring cleanse may also be beneficial:

Cleavers spring tonic

Add a handful of fresh cleavers (*Galium aperine*) to a litre of spring water (you can use sparkling or still depending on your preference). Leave in the fridge overnight. Drink one bottle daily for a week to cleanse and support the lymphatic system.

Common collarette signs

A prominent white collarette can indicate that the person is suffering with irritable bowel syndrome or another stress-related condition. It implies that there is inflammation in the bowel, and if the collarette is jagged, it may also indicate that there is an issue with peristalsis caused by tension.

A very thin or almost invisible collarette may indicate that the person is lacking in digestive enzymes and may have difficulty absorbing nutrients from their food.

Protuberances or many crypts inside the boundary of the collarette may indicate pockets in the bowel (as with diverticulitis) or a predisposition to parasites.

A collarette which balloons outwards away from the pupil indicates slack muscle tone and poor function *at that point.*

The angle of fuchs is a collarette which is very pronounced. It almost looks like the sides of a mountain range rising up above the iris. This is often an indication of an over-active digestive system. There is a tendency towards fermentation, which causes gas to build up in the colon resulting in painful constipation. Inversion postures such as yoga shoulder stands or using an inversion board to relieve pressure on the area can be very helpful for clients displaying this sign, as can carminative herbs that relieve gas.

PART 9

Putting it all together—taking a case

W hen I set out to write this book, my goal was to attempt to make complex information easy for the average person to understand, as well as provide enough detail for informed healthcare practitioners to confidently put their knowledge into practice. The following section is designed to help you consolidate what you've learned so far, test yourself, and put all the pieces of the jigsaw together so you can make confident assessments which are really going to be helpful for yourself, or the person seeking your help.

Taking your first case

The only way to confidently take a case is to get started. Practice is key. The more eyes you look at, the more you will get a feel for which areas to focus on. As with any new endeavour, it's only with repeated practice that you will develop skill.

When you first start out, it's a good idea to practice taking a case with family and friends. You'll already have a good idea of their nature, personality, and probably some information about their health background. This will help you gain confidence that the information you glean from their iris is correct, as well as help you learn your way around.

There are some general guidelines which should be followed while you become familiar with taking a case with a person in front of you.

An important note of caution

A degree of sensitivity is always required when a person opens themselves up to the vulnerability of an iridology assessment. The key when taking a case is always to ask rather than tell.

It goes without saying that you must *never* frighten the person in front of you or make statements that cannot be backed up with what they have presented with. Iridology is not a parlour game and should only ever be used to reassure and empower—never to create fear or worry.

Careless words can cause untold worry. Ask questions. Take a detailed case history, and use this information to corroborate what the person is telling you with the corresponding signs visible from the eyes. This gives the patient confidence in what you are saying, as well as providing evidence for the root cause of their condition.

Remember we all have strengths and weaknesses and it is important to point out the positives alongside the negatives. As we have seen, iris signs relate to disposition, and may not currently be presenting as a health problem. Although it can be quite tempting when you first start out to mention some of the things you can see, it's wise to take your time before making any assessments. Clients are often very impatient to learn what you've observed; don't be coerced into making remarks which may or may not be relevant out of context.

My advice is always to schedule a follow up session so you have some time to go away, assess the health questionnaire, and consult your charts so you have time to put a thoughtful protocol together.

Where to start

The iris is rich with information; at first you may feel like there is too much information to take in. Don't get overwhelmed. Start with what you know.

Begin with the colour. Is the person a lymphatic type? Ask them about their skin. Are they prone to UTI infections or arthritic joints? Do they feel the cold?

Next move on to the fibre structure. Do they have a polyglandular daisy structure? If they are young women, ask them about their periods. If they are older, are they having issues with the menopause?

Don't be tempted to make guess work and make the sign fit, but use what you see to formulate your questions.

After you have worked through the basic information, consider how the body is functioning as a whole. How might the systems be impacting one another? For example, if there is a liver sign along with a central heterochromia, could liver function be impacting the way they break down their food? Do they have a healthy diet?

Like the engine of a car, all the parts must work together for things to run smoothly. You are the detective. There are many pieces of the puzzle that may not immediately be apparent—it's your job to put them all together.

If there are markings that don't seem to fit or you are unsure about, make a note of them for future reference. They may later prove significant.

Exercise: ask a friend

Ask someone you know well if you can take their case.

Before you look at their eyes, ask them to complete a short health questionnaire. If you are already a practitioner, use one you are familiar with in your clinical practice. If not, then take some time to think about the kinds of questions that would be most helpful in aiding your understanding of the person in front of you. As I have repeatedly said, iridology is not fortune telling—don't make it into a guessing game. Completing a short health questionnaire will give you some key areas to look out for and focus on.

The next step is obviously to take a look at the person's eyes. Begin by using a hand-held lens and following the instructions outlined in Part Two.

Make notes on the following observations:

1. What is the person's general disposition when they arrive for the appointment? E.g. are they anxious, tired, excitable?
2. Are there any obvious features you can observe with the naked eye; for example, dark circles under the eyes, yellowing of the sclera, dilated pupils, or cholesterol rings?

3. What colour are the eyes?
4. What observations can you make about their pupils?
5. How open/closed is the general structure?
6. Are there any obvious markings, such as lacunae or dark spots? What colour are they?
7. Which area of the body do these markings relate to on the iris chart?
8. Are there any gaps, lacuna, or rarefication? What reflex points do they relate to?
9. What intuitive impressions can you gain from the personality of the client that may impact their lifestyle choices or ability to make beneficial changes for their health?—This is obviously much easier when you know the person!
10. What dietary recommendations, lifestyle interventions, supplements, or herbal remedies might you recommend?

By regularly using this step-by-step process you're much less likely to feel overwhelmed and make useful observations about your patients.

Take some time to collate your information before arranging a time to check back with the person. Ask for their input into how accurate your findings were.

Always keep a record of your practice consultations so you can build up a portfolio of case studies you can refer back to in the future. You'll be pleasantly surprised by how quickly you get used to seeing patterns and learning how to change your questioning based on what you see.

PART 10

Case studies

The following section contains real-life cases (the names have been changed for confidentiality), which will hopefully help you get a feel for the amazing way that iridology can help you tune into your patients and create more refined individualised protocols that really get results.

Case study 1: Robin

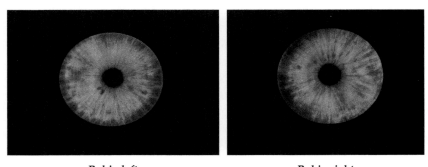

Robin left   **Robin right**

Background history

Robin is a fifty-year-old man seeking herbal support for indigestion, nausea, and feelings of lethargy, depression, and a lack of motivation.

On arriving at the appointment Robin appeared to be quite anxious, and a little bit overwhelmed. His alarm clock hadn't gone off in time for the appointment, and he had consequently arrived slightly late. He appeared to be quite flustered and was grateful for a cup of chamomile tea which helped him to relax.

As is my usual practice, I had previously asked Robin to complete a client intake form so I could compare my iris observations with his medical history. I often find that what clients list as their main health concerns on the form isn't always what they choose to discuss during the session. In this instance, this proved to be the case.

My first impression of Robin was that he was quite a worrier. We began immediately by discussing an ongoing situation with a work colleague who had recently been causing issues at his place of business. It was obvious this was something that had been really bothering him for quite some time, but he had kept it in, waiting for an opportunity to let off some steam.

He explained that they had both started in their new job at around the same time, and initially had become quite good friends. However, a few weeks ago, the colleague had created some problems within the department and laid some of the blame on Robin. This had placed quite a lot of strain on him, as he was keen to do well in this new job and wanted to be liked and respected. Although he had politely tried to distance himself from his co-worker, the colleague appeared unable to accept Robin's personal boundaries, and was telephoning him after work to discuss his numerous problems. The colleague's calls were leaving Robin feeling worried and frazzled.

On the one hand he felt a certain amount of loyalty to his colleague as they had both started work at the same time, but he was unable to speak up for himself and report the issue to his boss as he was worried it might reflect badly on him.

My initial opinion was that Robin appeared to be a kind and caring man who was a natural peacemaker. He wanted to be a people pleaser, and had tried his best to soothe over a difficult situation and move on. However, this approach hadn't worked and he had now reached a point whereby he dreaded going into work, and did not have the physical reserves to develop resilience to the prolonged stress.

As the session progressed, it was revealed that Robin had a history of gut-related issues that were usually triggered by stress. He would sometimes use alcohol to help him relax, but he felt that this coping mechanism was becoming much more of a regular habit than he would like, and it was only adding to his feelings of depression and anxiety. He had lost his appetite, and was mostly grabbing convenience food and sugary snacks to help keep him going throughout the day. This was causing him to experience indigestion, bloating and a feeling of being sick after eating. His GP had recently prescribed Omeprazole, (a medication used to treat indigestion, heartburn, and acid reflux,) but Robin was reluctant to take it as he felt this would only be masking the root cause of his problems, which he instinctively felt were related to his poor diet and the stress at work.

In the last few days, he had also noticed a recurrence of eczema, which he used to suffer with as a child. The last time he had experienced skin issues was during a stressful time at University when he was sitting exams and his father had died.

Robin described feeling very low for some time. He explained that he was unable to take too much adrenaline, or even listen to music. He felt vulnerable and over-sensitive to other people's negative emotions, and avoided watching too much television. He felt like all there was to see was drama and bad news, which only served to exacerbate his feelings of anxiety. He had heard about adrenal fatigue, and after reading about herbs on the internet, was hopeful a formula could help improve his mood and energy levels. He felt an urgent need to take action as he was becoming increasingly worried about getting ill, and how this might further affect his job if he had to take time off.

From our meeting together, I sensed that Robin was a very sensitive individual whose kind nature was often taken advantage of by others. He was a high-flying achiever who did not like to burden people with his problems, but he had reached a point of burnout and was in need of some support.

Iridology assessment

The silk constitution

This constitution is sometimes referred to as the "high resistance type.[48]" It was clear to me from our time together that Robin is the sort of person who would prefer to keep pushing on with life until he reached the point where he ran out of steam. From the outset it was obvious that Robin needed some nervous system support which included herbs to help him switch off and relax, as well as reduce the tension which was causing problems with his digestive system.

My first observation was that Robin had relatively small pupils, which as we have seen, can be an indication of over tense muscle tone and difficulty releasing emotions.[49] This was further evidenced by the nerve rings and radial contraction furrows visible in both eyes.[50]

In addition to both of these iris signs, his silk constitution indicated he was rather more used to keeping things in and solving his own problems than discussing them openly with others. Talking about a situation, which had been causing him distress for some time, had been quite challenging for him. As well as supporting him with some dietary advice, I felt it may also be worthwhile to signpost him to other adjunctive therapies such as mindfulness, yoga, or even some gentle exercise (he was currently doing nothing as he felt he didn't have the energy,) which would help to release the valve so he could let off some steam.

Collarette signs

It was unsurprising to hear that all of this stress was having a detrimental effect on Robin's digestive system, and that his predisposition to nervous tension and worry was affecting his appetite and ability to properly assimilate nutrients from the food he was eating. This was creating a catch-twenty-two situation. His reliance on sugar and alcohol to wind down was depleting his already over-worked adrenal glands. This meant he had even less energy or enthusiasm to devote time to preparing healthy meals.

---

[48] Refer to information on the silk constitution on Pg 45.
[49] Refer to information on pupil size on Pg 23–27.
[50] Refer to information on concentric rings and radial furrows on Pgs 71–73.

Notice the almost invisible collarette in these images. When the collarette is difficult to see or (sometimes almost non-existent,) this is an indicator that the person is at a natural disadvantage when it comes to the proper absorption and assimilation of nutrients. Although Robin knew he was feeling tired, this didn't make him slow down until he reached the point of exhaustion. His lack of appetite may even have been to avoid facing digestive issues which he knew would slow him down further to the point whereby he may even need to take time off work.

Pigmentation

Psoric spots

Some iridologists believe that psoric spots[51] indicate an emotional inability to learn life's lessons. It was clear talking to Robin that he tended to avoid confrontation and often allowed people to take advantage of his kindness, which he really resented.

According to Traditional Chinese Medical theory, suppressing the emotions "injures" the liver, and indeed we can see a large patch of brown pigmentation covering the liver spot at seven o'clock in the left iris.

Energetically, the liver has a major role to play when it comes to regulating our emotions. In today's fast paced society, liver qi stagnation (improper flow of energy to the organ)[52] is commonly found among people who are failing to maintain the proper, healthy work-life balance. This disruption of liver "qi" can lead to feelings of anger, anxiety, and depression. Physically, the liver is responsible (along with the spleen, gall-bladder and stomach) for regulating digestion.[53] One of its main functions is to produce bile, a fluid whose purpose is to break down fat from the food we eat. Poor liver function can therefore cause a ranger of gastrointestinal issues including nausea and a lack of appetite.

---

[51] Refer to information on Pg 73.
[52] Sarah Murphy, *Herbs and Liver Health,* 1st Edition, (Caernarfon: Wales, Herbary Books, 2020), 20.
[53] Murphy, *Herbs and Liver Health*, 10.

Other signs

There is also evidence of a scurf rim in the left eye (eight, nine, and eleven o'clock,) and in the right eye at (two, three, and four o'clock), which also provides us with some information around Robin's ability to eliminate. Compounded with the signs of a yellowish lymphatic rosary,[54] and his lymphatic constitution, this would explain the issues that Robin is currently having with his skin. With this in mind, it would be prudent to add some herbs which help him to clear metabolic waste products from the system in order to reduce his itching and eczema flare up. Energetically, being a very sensitive individual, it might also be beneficial for Robin to explore new ways to express his emotions in a healthy way.

Therapeutic interventions

We spent some time discussing Robin's diet and how we could make simple changes to increase his energy levels and mood. He agreed to try eating soothing porridge oats for breakfast, and to swap his regular morning coffee for a nerve building cup of herbal tea which I had made up for him. The tea was a blend of Vervain (*Verbena officinalis*), Lime flowers (*Tilia europea*) Rose petals (*Rosa* sp.), Hibiscus (*Hibiscus sabdariffa*), and Skullcap (*Scutellaria lateriflora*).

He later reported that he was enjoying this new morning ritual as it allowed him to take a few moments to relax in the morning, whereas before he had dreaded getting up and was therefore much more likely to be rushing around or late. This new routine allowed him to feel much more relaxed and prepared for the day.

Based on Robin's presentation, his case history and observations made from the iris, I prescribed the following combination of herbs in tincture form to be taken at the dosage of 5 ml twice daily, fifteen minutes before food. One dose was taken during his office breaktime at 11 am, and the second dose toward the end of the working day at around 3:30 pm. He looked forward to taking his medicine, and felt that it was soothing to know he had it with him during moments he felt unable to cope.

---

[54] Refer to information on Pgs. 7 & 74.

- Ashwagandha (*Withania somnifera*)
- Dandelion root (*Taraxacum officinale*)
- Chamomile (*Matricaria recutita*)
- Cramp bark (*Viburnum opulus*)
- Cardamom seed (*Elletaria cardamomum*)
- Gentian (*Gentiana lutea*)
- Liquorice root (*Glycyrrhiza glabra*)
- Ginger root (*Zingiber officinalis*)

The aim of the formula was to nourish the nervous system and reduce muscular spasm in the digestive tract. The prescription takes into account Robin's silk constitution which means he has a tendency to over-worry and push himself too hard. The cleansing, bitter herbs helped to support his lymphatic constitution, and clear out the build-up of metabolic waste in order to calm his eczema flare up and help him feel lighter.

Chamomile was added to support Robin's frazzled nervous system and provide gentle herbal support for his delicate digestion. Ashwagandha aided the action of chamomile, while at the same time pacifying his natural tendencies to worry. The addition of liquorice root helped to gently support Robin's over-worked adrenal glands, while ensuring there was adequate stomach acid to properly break down the food he was eating. The addition of very small amounts of cardamom and ginger served as warming messenger herbs to counteract the cold energy of the bitter herbs, as well as open up the channels to get the medicine to where it needed to go. The combined action of the carminative herbs helped ensure that food was being properly digested without discomfort or bloating.

As Robin is a sensitive individual, I wanted to start with a gentle formula to nurture and support him as he implemented some new dietary changes and got some rest. I'm pleased to say that three weeks later he came to see me again, looking vibrant and with much more energy. He commented that his work colleagues had made mention of how well he was looking, and that he attributed this to his prescription and his new morning routine. The herbs had also helped to rejuvenate his depleted nervous system to the point where he had finally plucked up enough courage to speak with his work colleague frankly about the ongoing situation. He arranged a meeting with his boss who had signposted him to some HR resources which had helped him begin the work of establishing healthy energetic boundaries, which made him feel much more in control of the situation, and life in general.

Case study 2: Violet

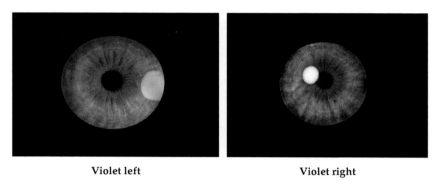

Violet left   **Violet right**

Background history

Violet is a forty-two-year-old digital marketer. She booked an appointment for support with her digestive health, and some issues she was having around transitioning into the menopause. She had recently been experiencing flare ups of IBS (irritable bowel syndrome), which generally manifested as constipation, but motions would become loose whenever she felt under pressure, or in the run up to her period.

At age sixteen, Violet had been diagnosed with Coeliac disease—an autoimmune condition in which the body attacks the digestive system when exposed to gluten. Over time, this had caused damage to the gut lining, meaning she was less able to derive nutrients from her food. Chronic malabsorption of vitamins and minerals had led to her becoming anaemic, and when not managed, caused her to feel very lethargic and in need of afternoon naps. As a self-employed person this was interrupting her daily work flow and causing her a great deal of frustration.

Her problems were exacerbated by the fact she had recently recovered from two bouts of Covid—each episode lasting for a period of about four weeks. The impact on her ability to work was causing her a great deal of stress. She was feeling overwhelmed by her workload, and felt compelled to work additional hours to make up for lost time.

Although Violet was very switched on when it came to her diet, she was finding that foods she used to be able to tolerate were now causing her issues. In addition, she had inexplicably put on weight, which made her feel even more sluggish and low.

Her medical history revealed that at age 21 she had contracted Giardia (a tiny parasite found on surfaces, or in soil, food, or water that has been contaminated with faeces from infected people or animals.) This is an extremely unpleasant disease that causes distressing digestive symptoms, including chronic diarrhea.

Violet had recently had a flare up of athlete's foot and an uncomfortable episode of thrush, both of which were made worse by the summer heat. Although she does not suffer from allergies, she was mildly asthmatic as a child. She felt that her recent brush with Covid had affected her breathing, which at times felt rather laboured. This meant she was unable to continue with her daily walks, which she had come to enjoy over the lockdown period.

In short, Violet was feeling demotivated and depressed. She was entirely fed up with the whole situation and in need of some dietary advice and herbal support to help her "get her powers back."

Iridology assessment

Mixed biliary constitution

Violet has a mixed constitution with a tendency towards the haematogenic (more brown than blue). This can clearly be seen in the photographs, which show a blue bottom layer, overlaid with a generalised brown diathesis, with emphasis around the digestive zone.

As we have seen, the colour brown (when overlaying the foundational base colour) indicates a tendency to accumulate toxic material in the corresponding area. In this case both the stomach, and small and large intestines are all affected, with "leakage"—also potentially impacting the tissues in the lung and chest area.

In mixed biliary constitutions, it is common for people to eat a healthy diet yet still experience digestive problems. This is because their inherited disposition means that the liver, gallbladder, and pancreas (which all play a part in stimulating biliary secretions such as stomach acid, saliva etc.) are often labouring under par. This means the body lacks the tools to adequately break down food. Regardless of how healthy the diet, this can lead to large undigested particles evading the body's checkpoints and getting into places they shouldn't technically go. This creates all manner of health issues, such as candidiasis (an overgrowth of a natural yeast that makes up part of the gut microflora), leaky gut syndrome, and other chronic digestive problems, which have a far-reaching impact, not just on the microbiome, but the entire physical body.

Violet's natural disposition may have been further thrown out of balance by her recent exposure to Covid. A year-long investigation was recently undertaken by experts at Cambridge University Hospitals (CUH) NHS Foundation Trust, Bedfordshire Hospitals NHS Foundation Trust, the University of Bedfordshire, and volunteer patients across both counties, in which it was discovered that after coming into contact with the virus, many Covid patients suffered a disruption in the ratio of friendly to unfriendly bacteria in the gut.[55] The technical term for this phenomenon is *dysbiosis*.

As Violet was already predisposed to a compromised digestive system (as noted from both her case history and iris examination), this inherent disharmony was further disrupted by her exposure to the virus. During the appointment, Violet mentioned that her issues with food intolerances and recent weight gain had worsened since having Covid, which would seem to fit with this theory.

Concentric rings

Violet came across as an extremely intelligent person whose main employment as a digital marketer meant she spent a great deal of time sitting at a desk and engaging in mostly non-physical work. The photographs clearly show deep furrows (both radial and concentric rings), which are an indication that she holds a lot of tension in her body and easily succumbs to stress.

Her nervous predisposition, lack of movement, and inability to release tension may also be impacting bowel motility. As we have seen, stress affects the parasympathetic nervous system which is responsible for rest, and most importantly, *digest*.

Because of the additional burden of the extra pressure from her workload; Violet had taken to eating at her desk and was not taking time out to have a proper break. Although she was preparing healthy

---

[55] Cook, David, "Friendly gut bacteria speeds long Covid recovery", December 1, 2021, *Cambridge University Hospitals NHS Foundation Trust*, https://www.cuh.nhs.uk/news/friendly-gut-bacteria-speeds-long-covid-recovery/

meals, the fact she was eating while on the go meant she was almost certainly not deriving maximum nutritional benefit from her carefully prepared meals.

Iris markings

A small, dark brown spot is visible at about 5 o'clock in the assimilation zone of the right iris. This marking lies is in the region of the pancreas. The pancreas has a dual role. It secretes hormones (like insulin and glucagon) that help the body to regulate blood sugar, and digestive enzymes (like lipase and amylase) that help the body break down fats and carbohydrates. Violet's case history in conjunction with this marking, is an indicator that herbs to help support the functioning of the pancreas may be helpful.

Therapeutic interventions

My first suggestion was to encourage Violet to start getting outdoors and moving more, even if it was only for ten minutes each day. Not only would taking a short break be helpful in reducing stress, the fresh air and movement would help oxygenate the blood and potentially increase uptake of iron absorption.

When questioned about her diet, it came to light that Violet was drinking a large glass of fruit smoothie for breakfast each morning. This is a lot of sugar for the pancreas to deal with in one hit, and was likely contributing to the energy slumps she was experiencing in the early afternoon. She was also using coffee for energy and was drinking up to four cups each day. We agreed that both the smoothies and the coffee had to go, and that a short ten-day gut rebalancing programme would be beneficial to give her digestive system a well-earned break.[56]

Along with the recommended dietary changes, I prescribed herbs and supplements that would help to reduce the number of unfriendly bacteria in the intestines and rebalance the microbiome. As studies have shown that certain blends of probiotics and prebiotics can also influence the severity and persistence of symptoms of post

[56] Sarah Donoghue, "10 Day Herbal Reset Programme", 2023. Alchemilla Apothecary. https://alchemilla.co/herb-store/10-day-herbal-detox/

COVID-19 infection.[57,58] I also prescribed a suitable blend, along with a gentle digestive enzyme formula to take some of the burden from the pancreas and digestive organs.

The following herbal prescription was dispensed:

Measured amounts of psyllium husks and bentonite clay taken in the form of a cleansing drink first thing in the morning on an empty stomach.[59] 5 ml of the following herbal tincture was to be taken at 11 am, and again at 3 pm.

- Chamomile (*Matricaria recutita*)
- Calendula (*Calendula officinalis*)
- Wormwood (*Artemisia absinthium*)
- Barberry (*Berberis vulgaris*)
- Thyme (*Thymus vulgaris*)
- Marshmallow root (*Althaea officinalis*)

Chamomile is an excellent herb for helping to rebalance the delicate microbiome. Studies have shown it has an anti-inflammatory, antispasmodic, antiviral, and anti-fungal effect, and that it is effective at combatting overgrowth of *Candida albicans*.[60,61]

Wormwood and barberry are bitter herbs that support the function of the liver, as well as stimulate the secretion of vital digestive enzymes.

Thyme is a warming herb which is supportive of both the digestive system and the lungs. I wanted to add something that would help balance the energy of the formula, as well as open up the lungs to improve oxygenation. On an energetic level, this aromatic herb also has the

---

[57] Robert Thomas et al., "A Randomised, Double-Blind, Placebo-Controlled Trial Evaluating Concentrated Phytochemical-Rich Nutritional Capsule in Addition to a Probiotic Capsule on Clinical Outcomes among Individuals with COVID-19" *The UK Phyto-V Study, COVID* 2, no. 4, (March 2022): 433–449, https://www.mdpi.com/2673-8112/2/4/31

[58] Cook, "Friendly gut speeds long COVID recovery," 2021.

[59] Full details for dosages and information about the 10-day detox protocol can be obtained from the author on request.

[60] Sima Sadat Seyedjavadi et al. "The Antifungal Peptide MCh-AMP1 Derived From *Matricaria chamomilla* Inhibits *Candida albicans* Growth via Inducing ROS Generation and Altering Fungal Cell Membrane Permeability", *Frontiers in microbiology*, 10, (January 2020): 3150. 21, doi:10.3389/fmicb.2019.03150

[61] Zahra Shiravani et al., "Chamomile Extract versus Clotrimazole Vaginal Cream in Treatment of Vulvovaginal Candidiasis: A Randomized Double-Blind Control Trial", *J Pharmacopuncture* 24, no. 4, (December 2021):191–195, doi: 10.3831/KPI.2021.24.4.191.

wonderful ability to lift the spirits, and nourish lung qi, something that Violet was very much in need of.

Calendula is a soothing, demulcent herb that also has an action against candida overgrowth.[62] Calendula is an excellent healer, and I often add it to formulas where there is evidence of potential leaky gut syndrome. Not only does it improve the general tone and integrity of the entire gut lining, it also helps to repair gaps in the tight junctions which stop undigested food particles from entering the gut. The soothing action of calendula was supported with the addition of marshmallow, which would sweeten the formula slightly and help take the edge of an otherwise rather pungent formula.

Shortly after the cleanse I received a message from Violet to say that she was feeling much better, and that the 10-day cleansed had opened her eyes to the fact that she had been running herself into the ground. She had booked a holiday and was planning to take some much-needed recuperation time to nurture herself. She had felt that the formula had been really beneficial, and was prescribed a repeat prescription to take away with her. She was pleased with her progress and the fact she had now gained some new tools with which to support herself should she begin to feel run down again in the future.

Case study 3: Fern

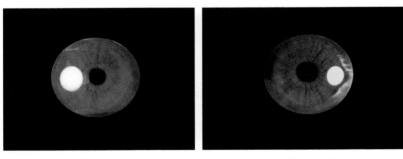

Fern left   Fern right

---

[62] Christopher Menzies-Trull, *Herbal Medicine—Keys to physiomedicalism including pharmacopoeia*, 2nd Edition, Newcastle: England, 2013.

Background history

Fern is a healthy, bright, thirty-year-old nutritional therapist. She was interested in booking an appointment to learn more about her individual constitution and how it could be better supported with diet and herbal supplementation.

She was currently happy and well, but had recently felt a little run down. This was very unusual for her as she sleeps well, manages stress by practicing yoga on a daily basis, and, being interested in nutrition, is very stringent about her diet. From time to time, she does enjoy sweets and chocolate, but keeps this to a minimum as a number of her family members have diabetes. Her energy levels are usually quite good, and so naturally she was a little concerned about why this might be happening.

Although generally well, she had made a visit to A&E in January after having the sensation she was unable to breathe. Prior to that she had a chronic cough and had been prescribed an inhaler by the GP. She described the sensation as not being able to get enough oxygen into her lungs. This had been followed up by a specialist, but no cardiovascular issues were found.

In recent months she had also experienced what she described as a "fluttering" sensation in her chest. Although infrequent, these episodes did make her worry about her heart.

Another health concern was her vision. As a therapist, she spends a lot of time in front of screens and feels that her glasses are not the right prescription. She was keen to look into any herbs that might be beneficial for her eyesight, as she felt this was exacerbating her tendency towards tension headaches.

Iridology assessment

Haematogenic constitution

Fern has a classic pure brown iris. Unlike the other types, even with an iriscope, it's very difficult to ascertain the fibre structure as the iris is deeply suffused with pigment. This feature is sometimes referred to as the *chromatophoric carpet*, as the chomatophore is the name of the cell that secretes this pigment.

Key indications for the pure brown iris are blood composition, high blood pressure, and circulatory issues. The fact that Fern is of also of an anxious disposition and regularly suffers with tension headaches is one reason why monitoring blood pressure may be prudent.

Crypts

Although a very minor, almost indiscernible feature, small crypts are visible in the lung area of each iris. In another individual these might be considered to be rather unimportant, however in a dense iris with no other gaps in the fibres, they may have more significance.

Venous ring

Although not as clear in the pictures, during our appointment I was able to see the beginnings of a slight venous ring around the outer edge of Fern's iris.

The venous ring is blue in colour and suggests sluggish circulation. When very pronounced, this can indicate there are issues around blood being carried back to the heart. People displaying this sign often have more difficulty cleansing waste products from the blood, which results in less absorption of oxygen. Inevitably, poor oxygenation of the tissues is the result. It is a common sign in older people with a haematogenic constitution.

Therapeutic interventions

For Fern, supporting the heart and enabling better oxygenation of the tissues was going to be important. I believed that this was the likely root cause of a number of her issues, including the low energy levels, palpitations, headaches, the visit to A&E, and the recent deterioration in her eyesight.

For this reason, the proposed herbal formula was focused around herbs to support the proper functioning of the circulatory system, and strengthening the heart muscles. In addition, I added some gentle nervines to reduce the potential for high blood pressure, and her natural tendency towards anxiety.

With this in mind, the following prescription was dispensed, to be taken 5 ml three times daily.

- Hawthorn berries (*Crataegus monogyna*)
- Bilberry (*Vaccinium myrtillus*)
- Lime blossom (*Tilia europea*)
- Motherwort (*Leonorus cardiaca*)
- Yellow dock (*Rumex crispus*)
- 2 drops of facing heaven chilli tincture (*Capsicum anuum*)

I potentized the above-mentioned formula with Elm Bach flower remedy. Fern is a highly skilled nutritional practitioner who does in fact have an excellent grasp on her own constitution and how to look after herself. However, her lack of confidence in her own abilities was a stumbling block when it came to knowing which approach was best. Instead of working with her constitution, she was over worrying about each individual sign and symptom, which had left her feeling overwhelmed about which approach to take.

In addition to the herbal support, I also recommended she try including some inverted yoga positions into her daily practice. I also wanted her to include more garlic in her food, as well as some supplements to nourish the blood. At this point Fern did mention that she was already taking spirulina as she had read it was similar in chemical composition to haemoglobin.

I'm pleased to report that Fern did not feel the need for a follow up appointment. She said the session had given her the confidence to follow her intuitions when it came to looking after her own health, although she did appreciate that even therapists sometimes have to seek objective advice when it comes to trying to treat oneself. Good advice indeed.

Exercise: take your first case!

Iridology is not fortune telling. The study of the iris, when made alongside accurate case taking, and perhaps other diagnostic tools, such as looking at the tongue and feeling the nature of the pulse, is a very valuable addition to the practitioner's repertoire. If done sensitively, it can engage the client in a way that fosters a connection with the practitioner, and in many cases allows them to open up and offer information they may not initially have volunteered.

It can be a daunting prospect to take your first case. Be confident that asking simple questions to verify your observations is a really good way to engage your patient, in a way that makes them feel you are paying attention to them as an individual, and that you are going the extra length to personalise their treatment. Have confidence and have a go. Practice really is the best way to learn.

Checklist

1. Are there any obvious *medically recognised* signs that indicate the person may need conventional support from their GP?

2. Define the constitution from the general colour of the iris.
3. Look at the general fibre structure—e.g. are they a silk or a hessian type?
4. What does the fibre structure tell you about the state of the person's nervous system? How resilient are they?
5. Check for gaps in the fibre structure, or areas where the fibre structure is particularly dense in comparison to the rest of the iris. Which areas of the body do these observations correlate to on the iris chart?
6. Are there any particular markings such as pigmentation, dark spots? What colour are they? Locate them on the iris chart and ask about the corresponding organ systems.
7. Are there any crypts? Can you spot any areas of rarefication?
8. Is there a central heterochromia? What colour is it? Use this information to enquire about the digestive system.
9. What other colours, patterns, and markings can you identify in the iris? If you're unsure, make a note of these for future reference.
10. Based on the information you have gleaned, along with the person's case history, what suitable recommendations might you make based on their current lifestyle, diet, and constitutions? What therapeutic interventions might you suggest? What supplements or herbs may be beneficial? Do they need to be referred to another specialist practitioner?

CONCLUSION

It is my fervent belief that we still have a lot to learn about the mysteries of the human body. It may well be that the eye holds many more secrets to our inner workings than we could ever have imagined.

Iridology it seems, is not a universal language, with many different schools offering varying interpretations of what they are seeing before them. Taking this view means that in its current phase, iridology truly is in the eye of the beholder, and in this respect, can still be viewed as a pioneering study with much left to discover.

With the advent of new photographic technology and digital analysis software, combined with the increasing interest in this subject, it is my ardent hope that serious work will continue in this field, allowing us to better serve our patients and encourage people to seek nature's wisdom to create balance and harmony in our busy, modern lives. It is only through education and the sharing of this knowledge that we can feel we are not at the mercy of the wind when it comes to looking after our own health.

I strive to play a small part in this important work and am forever indebted to the many patients who have passed through my doors with an open mind and willingness to embark on this journey with me.

GLOSSARY

Central heterochromia: A defined area of pigmentation (can be brown, yellow, or white) that appears around the pupil and extending out into the collarette. Depending on the colour, this can indicate a variety of potential health concerns in the digestive system, including under-activity of gastric secretions, and lowered function of the liver, gallbladder and pancreas. From the Latin *hetero* (different) and *chromia* (colour).

Chronic: Long term pathology. Associated with dark signs in the iris.

Collarette: The frilly rope like structure located about a third of the way out towards the edge of the iris. Sometimes referred to as the *autonomic neve ring* or the *pupillary ruff*.

Constitution: The natural disposition a person is born with. The constitution can be considered a person's natural "make-up", which is determined at birth, dictated by genetics, and influenced by environmental and lifestyle factors.

Contraction furrows: Circular grooves appearing in a concentric pattern. Caused by prolonged contraction of the dilator muscles, these are an indication of an overactive nervous system, mineral deficiencies, or metabolic imbalances. In some books they are referred to as "nerve rings."

Crypt: Holes in the iris structure, often diamond shaped. Usually indicates a long standing degenerative or chronic condition in the corresponding zone. Many small crypts located inside the boundary of the collarette and stomach zone may indicate a tendency towards parasites.

Diathesis: The iris "overlay."

Haematogenic: Pertaining to brown pigmentation of the iris. Persons with a haematogenic constitution have brown eyes.

Lacuna: A hole appearing in the texture of the iris. Can be open or closed. Larger than crypts, they come in variety of shapes, and indicate inherited signs of energy insufficiency in the corresponding zone.

Lymphatic rosary: A ring of tophi or spots in the outer iris zone. Usually associated with the lymphatic constitution.

Miasm: A weakness or mark left behind after physical disease which can be transmitted down the generational chain.

Mixed biliary: Persons with a mixture of blue and brown eyes (lymphatic and haematogenic constitutions.)

Pinguecula: Deposits of yellow or clear fatty tissue visible on the sclera, usually attributed to poor fat metabolism.

Radial furrow: A crease in the iris tissue which usually begins at the outer edge of the pupil and extends to the outer edge of the iris. Sometimes referred to as "wagon wheel spokes."

Rarefaction: An area in the iris in which the fibres appear to be less dense or even missing. This is a sign of general weakness in that area, for which long-term, supportive measures are usually required.

Sclera: The white tissue around the iris commonly referred to as the eyeball.

Scurf rim: A dark zone in the outer portion of the iris. Usually an indication of poor elimination via the skin.

BIBLIOGRAPHY

Akers, Matthew, director. *Marina Abramovic: The Artist is Present,* Show of Force, 2012. Film.

British Thyroid Foundation. "Thyroid Eye Disease." Revised 2021. "https://www.btf-thyroid.org/thyroid-eye-disease-leaflet"

Colton, James and Sheelagh Colton, *Iridology—Health Analysis & Treatments from the Iris of the Eye,* UK: Element books, 1996.

Cook, David. "Friendly gut bacteria speeds long Covid recovery." Published December 1, 2021. *Cambridge University Hospitals NHS Foundation Trust.* https://www.cuh.nhs.uk/news/friendly-gut-bacteria-speeds-long-covid-recovery/

Deck, Joseph. *Fundamentals of Iridology.* 1st Edition. Etlingen: Self-published, 1965.

Donoghue, Sarah. "10 Day Herbal Reset Programme" 2023. *Alchemilla Apothecary.* https://alchemilla.co/herb-store/10-day-herbal-detox/

Guild of Naturopathic Iridologists International. "The History of Iridology." Published Jan 2023, https://www.gni-international.org/the-history-of-iridology/

Hall, Dorothy. *Iridology.* London: Piatkus, 1994.

Jackson-Main, Peter, *Practical Iridology.* London: Carroll & Brown, 2004.

Karamanou, Marianna, Charalambos Vlachopoulos, Christodoulos Stefanadis & George Androutsos. "Professor Jean-Nicolas Corvisart des Marets (1755–1821): Founder of modern cardiology." Last modified 2010. *Hellenic Journal of Cardiology: HJC / Hellēnikē kardiologikē epitheōrēsē.* 51 (2010):290–3.

Ledoux, Danielle. "Vision and Down Syndrome." Published 2022. *National Down Syndrome Society.* https://ndss.org/resources/vision-down-syndrome

Lennon, John *"Aisumasen (I'm Sorry)."* Recorded July–August 1973. Track 3, side 1 on *Mind Games.* Apple, 1973, vinyl.

Mayo Clinic. "Graves' disease—Patient care & health information" 2022. *Mayo Foundation for Medical Education and Research (MFMER).* https://www.mayoclinic.org/diseases-conditions/graves-disease/symptoms-causes/syc-20356240

Menzies-Trull, Christopher. *Herbal Medicine —. Keys to physiomedicalism including pharmacopoeia, 2nd Edition.* Newcastle: England, 2013.

Munjal, Akul and Evan J. Kaufman. *Arcus Senilis.* Treasure Island (FL): StatPearls Publishing, 2022.

Murphy, Sarah. *Herbs and Liver Health, 1st Edition.* Caernarfon: Wales, Herbary Books, 2020.

The National Library of Medicine. "Jaundice Causes" 2022. https://medlineplus.gov/ency/article/007491.htm

O'Brian, Betty S., *The Core Curriculum Iris Analysis Manual,* 1st Revision. USA: Self-Published, 2016.

Ohsawa, George. *Macrobiotics—An Invitation to Health & Happiness, 6th Edition.* California: George Ohsawa Macrobiotic Foundation, 1984.

Pike, Helena. "Iridology—One science or many?" *The Guild of Naturopathic Iridologists International.* Published December 2, 2018. https://www.gni-international.org/iridology-one-science-or-many-new-research/

Pollington, Stephen. *Leechcraft—Early English Charms, Plantlore & Healing.* Cambridgeshire: Anglo-Saxon Books, 2011.

Postolache, Lavinia, and Cameron F. Parsa. "Brushfield Spots and Wölfflin Nodules Unveiled in Dark Irides Using Near-Infrared Light." *Scientific Reports* 8, no. 1 (2018). https://doi.org/10.1038/s41598-018-36348-6.

Seyedjavadi, Sima Sadat et al. "The Antifungal Peptide MCh-AMP1 Derived From *Matricaria chamomilla* Inhibits *Candida albicans* Growth via Inducing ROS Generation and Altering Fungal Cell Membrane Permeability." *Frontiers in microbiology* 10, (January 2020): 3150. doi:10.3389/fmicb.2019.03150

Shiravani Z, et al. "Chamomile Extract versus Clotrimazole Vaginal Cream in Treatment of Vulvovaginal Candidiasis: A Randomized Double-Blind Control Trial." *J Pharmacopuncture* 24, no. 4 (December 2021):191–195. doi: 10.3831/KPI.2021.24.4.191.

Schlegel, Emil. *Die Augendiagnose des Dr. Ignaz von Péczely*, 1887. Reprint, Antique Reprints, reprinted January 5th 2016.

Thomas, Robert, et al. "A Randomised, Double-Blind, Placebo-Controlled Trial Evaluating Concentrated Phytochemical-Rich Nutritional Capsule in Addition to a Probiotic Capsule on Clinical Outcomes among Individuals with COVID-19" *The UK Phyto-V Study, COVID* 2, no. 4, (March 2022): 433–449. https://doi.org/10.3390/covid2040031

Treben, Maria., *Health Through God's Pharmacy*. 22nd Edition. "Steyer: Austria, Wilhelm Ennsthaler, 1994."

White, Désirée and& Montserrat Rabago-Smith. "Genotype-phenotype associations and human eye colour" *Journal of Human Genetics*. 56, (October 2011); 5–7. https://doi.org/10.1038/jhg.2010.126

FURTHER READING & RESOURCES

Professional associations

The Guild of Naturopathic Iridologists International (GNI) is the leading body for iridologists in the UK. It also accepts members from overseas who have completed a certified course.

Established in 1994, this non-profit organisation was founded with the primary aim of providing the public with a register of qualified and professionally regulated Iridology practitioners. It offers member support, information and educational opportunities.

Information about their code of conduct, affiliated courses and list of registered practitioners can be found on their website: www.gni-international.org

Certified training courses

UK

The following courses are recognised by the Guild of Naturopathic Iridologists (GNI)

- Cambridge Holistic Iridology: https://thenaturalcentre.com/holistic-iridology/
- The College of Naturopathic Medicine: https://www.naturopathy-uk.com/courses-eu/courses-iridology/
- Holistic Health College London: www.holistichealthcollege.com
- UK College of Clinical Iridology: https://www.bcma.co.uk/clinical-iridology

The author also offers short introductory courses and workshops for interested enthusiasts online and at various locations throughout the UK. Information about upcoming workshops can be found on her website: www.alchemilla.co and in her weekly newsletter https://theherbalistsdiary.substack.com/

Information about her 10-day bowel cleansing and gut rebalancing programme is also available on the website.

The author can be contacted by sending an email enquiry to sarah@alchemilla.co

USA

My good friend and mentor Betty Sue O'Brian offers a number of professional iridology courses, details of which can be found at www.iridologyacademy.org

Courses are also available from The International Iridology Practitioner's Association: https://www.iridologyassn.org/

Iridology equipment

- Tony Miller offers courses and has a well stocked online shop at https://www.iridologyonline.com/
- Irislab.com also has professional iridology equipment for sale

Herbal suppliers and resources in the UK

Napiers

An independent herb shop, and one of the oldest suppliers of botanical products in the UK. They have been selling high quality herbal products for over 162 years. Their reputation and customer service are second to none.

18 Bristol Place, Edinburgh, EH1 1EZ. Telephone: 0131 225 5542. Email enquiries via website.

Baldwins

One of London's oldest and most established herbalists, supplying an extensive range of herbs, essential oils, and natural remedies online.

They are located at 171–173 Walworth Rd, London SE17 1RW. Telephone: 020 7703 5550 Email: sales@baldwins.co.uk

The Organic Herb Trading Company

For forty years the Organic Herb Trading Company has grown, sourced and supplied the UK's largest range of high-quality botanicals for a diverse range of customers in the herbal tea, food, skincare and medicinal markets. They have a worldwide customer base ranging from individuals to holistic healthcare practitioners. All their products are certified organic by the Soil Association.

Located at HQ—Butts Way, Milverton, Somerset TA4 1ND, UK. Telephone (0) 1823 401205. Email: info@organicherbtrading.com

Further resources

More information about rayid iridology can be found at https://rayid.com/iris-patternsstructures/

Iris charts

https://thenaturalcentre.com/shop/iridology-chart/

This is the chart originally created by Peter Jackson-Main, who very kindly allowed me to reproduce it in this book. This is the chart I was personally taught to use as a student. I highly recommend this high-quality resource, as well as Peter's book, which has formed the foundation of my own work.

Alternative iris charts

https://www.iridologyonline.com/charts
https://eyology.com/
https://iridology.com/product/universal-iridology-chart/

GRATITUDE

I am very fortunate indeed to be surrounded by some incredibly amazing individuals, without whom this project would not have been possible. My deepest gratitude must be expressed for the help and unconditional support of the following:

My fabulously knowledgeable and inspiring mentor Peter Jackson-Main, who has not only generously shared his sound herbal wisdom and advice with me for the last thirteen years, has also been a pillar of support for myself and my family for many more. I am deeply grateful for his kindness in allowing me to share his charts for this publication, and for his kind support of my work.

To Betty Sue O'Brian, for so benevolently sharing both her personal photographs and professional insights, offering advice and suggestions whenever asked. You are beyond gracious.

To Sharn Nulty-Harper, herbal friend and mentor extra-ordinaire, who is always has time for my herbal quandaries. I am truly indebted to you for your friendship and sage advice.

To my newest herbal mentor Lucy Jones, for giving me the courage to get out there and write a book—even if it does mean putting my head above the parapet! Likewise, to Monica Wilde, who by her unswerving enthusiasm for life has always inspired bravado and a "just do it!" attitude.

To V Harrigan for her many years of friendship, camaraderie, support and love, and to her daughter Elodie Harrigan, without whom it would not have been possible to source the stunning photographs for this book.

To my wonderful patients (especially those who were so generous in sharing their case studies, and personal stories.) I continue to learn so much from you every single day.

To the hard-working folks at Newquay Orchard who are always on the look out for ways to help raise the profile of herbal medicine in our community, and who have supported this project from the get-go.

Most of all I have to be thankful for my family who have always supported me on my herbal journey, throughout all its many ups and downs. Particular thanks go to my gorgeous husband Phillip who has endured many frustrating hours listening to me tapping away at the computer on our days off, helping me to maintain the belief it would all be worth it in the end.

INDEX